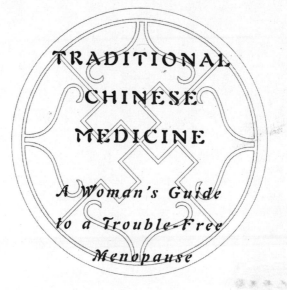

TRADITIONAL CHINESE MEDICINE

A Woman's Guide to a Trouble-Free Menopause

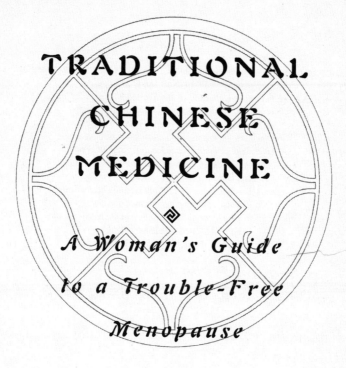

TRADITIONAL CHINESE MEDICINE

A Woman's Guide to a Trouble-Free Menopause

NAN LU, O.M.D., L.AC.,

with Ellen Schaplowsky

HarperResource

An Imprint of HarperCollinsPublishers

FIRST EDITION

Library of Congress Cataloging-in-Publication Data has been applied for.
ISBN 0-380-80904-4

00   01   02   03   04   RRD   10   9   8   7   6   5   4   3   2   1

*To my many extraordinary masters who have
gifted me with the deep knowledge and spirit
of true healing.*

*To my family—my parents and sisters,
my wife, Ling Shou, and my children,
Christina and Alicia*

—NAN LU

*To Nan Lu for his extraordinary ability
to create light wherever he goes;
To my son, Ian, my sister, Pat, and brothers
Michael, Tom, Jim, and Peter;
to my extended family, dear friends, and
Qigong sisters and brothers*

—ELLEN SCHAPLOWSKY

CONTENTS

PART TWO: GETTING TO THE ROOT CAUSE

PART THREE: HOW YOU CAN UNLOCK TCM'S ANCIENT SECRETS FOR A NATURAL, HORMONE-FREE MENOPAUSE

◈

MENOPAUSE:
The Last Great Opportunity to Prepare Yourself for a Long, Healthy Life

*M*ANY of my Western patients and my Qigong students like to joke with me. They say, "What did you do in your past life that you now have responsibility for helping so many women—especially those who are dealing with menopausal symptoms?" They're correct in the fact that about 95 percent of my patients are Western women. They're also correct when they point out that most of them fall into the thirty-five to fifty-five age range. I'm not sure what I did (good or bad!) in a past life, but I know in this life that each of my patients is very special to me. I feel privileged to bring unique healing knowledge to these women who are about to enter what could well be the most rewarding and spiritually liberating time of their lives. What I also love is how eager they are to pass this information along to the other women in their life. It's as if they've discovered a real hidden treasure.

The good-hearted teasing of my patients and students started me thinking about what else I could do to help Western women who need relief from health conditions that traditional Chinese medicine, or TCM as it is called, has treated successfully for thousands of years. For some reason or other (the ancient Chinese would call it fate), I have received ancient knowledge, or what we call the keys to special understanding, from one of my masters that can really help women who are going through one of the biggest, if not the biggest, transition of their lives. To one degree or another, the women I work with come away with a very different understanding of menopause that is highly rewarding and empowering of their whole being. So, I realized that what I really can do in the service of TCM is help as many women understand as deeply as possible the richness that the transition of menopause offers them.

From the ancient knowledge I've received from my master, I have come to understand that menopause represents the last great opportunity for a woman to prepare her body, mind, and spirit for a long, healthy life. Why? During this period, there is an enormous energy shift within a woman's body that goes far beyond physical changes. This shift, while profound, is natural and normal; it has the power to affect the mind, emotions, and spirit of those who pass through it. If a woman is able to understand this special opportunity and takes the time to readjust or strengthen her internal Qi (pronounced CHEE), then she can help prevent new problems arising from this energy transition. Otherwise, after this turning point, without a sufficient level of internal Qi, she will not have the power she needs to ward off the many health problems that often come with age.

I tell my patients to think of this time as preparation for a long car trip across the desert. This is their last great chance to make sure that their car is properly tuned, that it's full of gas or energy, and that they are rested enough to manage the drive. If you can take care of yourself very well during this transitional time, you can contain or even eliminate long-standing health issues and prevent new ones from developing.

THE TCM VIEW OF MENOPAUSE

Before we go much further, I would like to give you an idea of how TCM looks at the condition we in the West call menopause. It may interest you to know that "menopause" is a word that is not in the

TCM vocabulary. In ancient medical texts, menopause does not even appear. What does appear are many of the symptoms relating to women who reach this transitional age.

Menopause is basically a Western concept. TCM recognizes menopausal symptoms as Menstrual Cycle Ending Symptoms. In other words, TCM recognizes that the menstrual cycle has a beginning and it has an end. This is nature's way. Along this continuum, a woman may experience a variety of different problems if she is not healthy. If she is healthy, her menstruation will be problem-free. Menopause symptoms occur at the end of this natural cycle. Again, if a woman's menstrual cycle has been regular and mostly without problems, she should not experience a difficult menopause, unless outside factors such as stress, poor diet, lack of rest, etc., unbalance her system.

TCM has extensive experience in treating the entire spectrum of menstrual cycle symptoms. Today, in the medical texts used in all TCM medical colleges, there are twenty-two specific menstrual cycle symptoms. These include conditions such as delayed periods, early periods, fever during cramps, cold sores during the menstrual cycle, breast tenderness and pain during menstruation, premenstrual syndrome (PMS), or even specific kinds of menstrual headaches, among others. Interestingly, only one of the twenty-two symptoms relates to what we call menopause. This is the abovementioned Menstrual Cycle Ending Symptoms—the last set of problems a woman can have with her menstrual cycle before it ceases entirely.

Menstrual Cycle Ending Symptoms is then what we in the West call menopausal symptoms. From the TCM perspective, if a woman doesn't suffer from menstrual irregularities during a lifetime of cycles, it is highly unlikely that she will experience any symptoms during her last cycles. This brings us to the concept of prevention—a unique specialty of TCM and one of its most important principles.

I help many Western women address their menopausal symptoms. Most of the women I see have not taken very good care of themselves, even though many of them believe they have. I try to help them understand that this is really their last great opportunity to become truly healthy. I try to educate them about what they can do to eliminate, or substantially reduce, their current health problems and become stronger so that they can prepare their bodies for the years ahead. These are years that should be happy and healthy ones, during which women can flourish in so many ways. I tell them that menopause is a very real gateway that offers them a chance for renewal of their bodies, minds, and especially their spirits. Once again, I emphasize that prevention is the real key.

The journey after menopause takes us to the end of our mission in this plane of existence. I remind my patients that this journey can be a long, happy, and vibrant one, if they're well prepared. And, the most interesting aspect of it for Western women, I believe, is that this journey can be taken without hormone therapy.

While TCM has understood and treated the fundamental conditions of menopause, especially kidney Qi deficiency, for thousands of years, it may surprise you to know that TCM does not make a big deal of menopause. Why? Because TCM views menopause as part of the natural transition that all people—women and men —must go through as they grow older. No one is immune to the process of aging. The women I see for menopause always seem so relieved when I mention that men go through their own kind of menopause. It seems in the West that so much is made out of female menopause, that male menopause is almost never discussed. But, I can assure you that men too go through all kinds of mental, physical, emotional, and spiritual changes because everyone is under natural law and everyone must face the challenges of aging. While most people can't control the fact that they age, everyone can control how healthy they are as they do.

Many of my patients ask me: "Why do some people have such a difficult menopause and suffer from so many different problems?" I tell them that their problems are not the result of menopause, but the condition of their bodies before the transition gets underway. Simply put, as the body ages, its energy or Qi reserves decline naturally. You have less and less energy to do the same things. If you don't recalibrate your system for this energy differential, it will begin to take its toll and affect all your other organs. How badly it affects them is determined by how out of balance you are. The one organ it affects next for virtually all women is the liver. Why? Because the liver controls the smooth flow of all things in the body—blood, Qi, and emotions.

TCM believes that everyone is born with the ability to self-heal. TCM also appreciates that women, because of their menstrual cycle and their special organs—the uterus and ovaries—have a unique capacity for healing themselves and helping their bodies restore healthy functioning. This is an important point because it is this ability that allows women to alleviate symptoms of menopause—for good—without hormone therapy. TCM believes that healthy women have the capacity to make enough estrogen for their entire life. The estrogen level will not be as high as it was during a woman's childbearing years, but the amount of estrogen will be enough to last the rest of her life.

But, symptoms or no symptoms, TCM views menopause as the last great healing opportunity in a woman's life. And, TCM can offer the tools and techniques necessary to navigate this last great passage.

My message is simple: Embrace the unique and magnificent transition of menopause and take the time to learn how to care for yourself today so that all your tomorrows are filled with good health, not with debilitating conditions such as heart disease, osteoporosis, breast cancer, or other health-robbing problems. I would like to help you reawaken the self-healing gift that you were born with.

My goal is also simple: I want to share with you time-tested knowledge that has successfully helped literally millions and millions of Chinese women for many thousands of years and continues to do so today. Right now, thousands of Western women are beginning to benefit from this ancient knowledge. I want to help you understand why and how this natural transition of menopause occurs and help you learn how to apply TCM's time-

xvi 🔲   Introduction

tested wisdom for your own healing. I would like you to benefit from this information starting right now.

In my practice, my work is not just directed at treating the presenting condition (no matter what it is), but rather its aim is to help my patients learn how they became unwell in the first place, what the true root cause of their health problems is, and teach them how to take care of their body, mind, and spirit. In that concept, of course, TCM includes emotions. In the case of menopause, I try to help my patients realize that one of the biggest factors aggravating their health is chronic stress and anger. This is not only relevant to menopause, but also relates to the root cause of breast cancer. I also help educate my patients on the essential role eating for health plays in a smooth menopausal transition. The Chinese like to say: "You eat for someone else's stomach." Why? Because many people, especially in Western cultures where the food is plentiful, interesting, and delicious, select items that make their mouths feel good, but in reality, are damaging to the healthy functioning of their major organs.

We shall see in the information on food in Chapter 15 that this concept of eating for healing goes much deeper than the scientific aspect of foods such as calories, nutritional properties, vitamins, and such. It gets at the very essence of certain foods and which organs they can help heal. I urge you to pay particular attention to this ancient knowledge about foods and their healing properties. In my opinion, it is essential that all women learn how to eat for health, healing, and building Qi—particularly women who are entering perimenopause and those going through menopause. This is one daily activity where you have maximum control over making positive contributions to your health.

Even though I've been privileged to work with many masters who have passed to me tremendous secret healing skills for pain and sports injury, (especially sports injury), and even though I have practiced the martial arts since I was a child, it seems that the Universe has other things in mind for me. It has charged me with the mission of working with women, particularly those in the Western cultures, so that I can share what I know. The rewards for me have been great and the women I've met and helped even greater.

If you have picked up this book, chances are that you or someone you know is experiencing some phase of menopause, what we've seen TCM considers one of the two most important transitions in a woman's life. The time of pregnancy through childbirth is the first opportunity for a woman to transform her health. From my experience, I can see that many Western women missed this first chance to change. Along the way, they also accumulated new health problems, which cause their current menopausal difficulties. Unfortunately, with Western society's emphasis on youthful looks and staying young, menopause in our culture today carries a lot of baggage. And while there is nothing wrong with wishing to remain vibrant and healthy as we age, there is everything wrong with wishing to go against the natural law of the Universe and artificially maintain menstruation long after its natural life cycle should have ended.

Many women approach this time in their lives with fear, anxiety, and anger. There are so many factors responsible for this: there's the worry about heart disease, breast cancer, and osteoporosis. There's also the fear of growing old and possibly useless or incapacitated, and so many more negative thoughts that it's understandable that women have a difficult time maintaining a positive outlook through this transition. Part of my job is to help women understand that their thoughts are far more powerful and have far more energy than their actions. In my role as a healer, I must help them learn how to transform fear, worry, anxiety, and anger into powerful healing tools. I would also like to do this for you. Hope, peacefulness, and confidence in your own healing ability (an amazing gift with which you were born!) can help you make profound changes in your life.

Change can mean many things. TCM likes to think of this change as a time for new beginnings. You are at an age when your wisdom and experience should be respected. You have nothing to stop you from shedding old ways and discovering new and unexplored paths. This transition gives you a unique opportunity—a chance to reevaluate your whole being and your whole life. It is a time when you can nourish your spiritual side and begin to appreciate what is unique about you and your mission on earth. Never again will you be in a position to make such a quantum leap forward in your health and healing.

As we've said, one way to think about this period of your life is to see it as a long journey across the country for which you now have the planning responsibility. There are a variety of options you can choose. You can set off on a course that lets you take the interstate highways; these are familiar roads and will definitely get you to your destination in a predictable way. Or, you can decide to try a more interesting route that takes you along some local roads that you might never have seen had you not taken the time to plan this very special journey. This way lies more excitement and more of the unknown. Away from the monotonous hum of the interstate, you might find intriguing people, family stores, terrific restaurants, amazing landmarks, out-of-the-way museums, and other unexpected treasures and experiences. If you're unmarried, you might even stop and find the person of your dreams!

In other words, by addressing this change and approaching this turning point with optimism, enthusiasm, and a sense of purpose, your whole life can start to change. It can become deeper, richer and more fun than you ever imagined. Remember, the end point is the same for each of us. When our journey's over, it's the body's time to die.

TCM believes the spirit lives forever . . . enriched by this life's work. I've noticed in this country that there is a great deal of discomfort with discussing the end of life. But, the end is as natural as the beginning. It gives meaning to the need for spirituality in our lives, to go beyond the material and contact that eternal spark that is inside all of us. Though some of my patients are uncomfortable at first with this concept, if I can get them to accept the wonder of this amazing transition, they tell me that their life has become better than they ever thought possible.

Of course, you also have the option of continuing on with your old life. You can start hormone replacement therapy and keep going as if nothing has changed. You can have face peels and get face-lifts. You can take vitamins and try to take off pounds. You can continue on with your ten-hour workdays and two-hour workouts. But, the truth is, as you enter menopause, you are about to be immersed in an inner sea-change of far-reaching spiritual, emotional, and physical consequences. Are you going to let fear prevent you from flourishing? Or, are you going to embrace this opportunity and open a door to a whole new life—one that is healthy and sustainable over the wonderfully interesting time you have allotted to you?

I urge you to let yourself fully explore this unique opportunity so that you can make the best choice for you. I believe that for women in Western cultures, TCM can represent the local route described above. However, while this book can lead you up to the door of TCM, it is your responsibility to open the door and examine what is on the other side. Some women might be afraid to try TCM because they've been told that there are health risks associated with not taking hormone replacement therapy (HRT). Remember you are not the first person to try this natural healing path. For thousands of years, millions of women have chosen this path and discovered a natural, healthy way to complete their life's journey.

Remember also that TCM is not a basket full of "New Age" therapies. The time-tested nature of this medical system should help reassure you of its efficacy and effectiveness. Before we continue, it is important to point out that TCM is more than five thousand years old, and that practitioners of authentic TCM have been treating menopause naturally and its related symptoms successfully for many, many centuries. In describing this time of a woman's life, ancient Chinese texts say that as the door to one's childbearing years is closing, a new door is literally opening.

TCM recognizes that during the years leading up to menopause and in the years after, the body's energy system is undergoing a natural predictable, yet major, cyclical change. As a woman's Qi or vital energy alters, she is given this special opportunity we've discussed to transform herself. Far from being a time of barrenness, decline, and uselessness, TCM sees it as a deeply rewarding and rich opportunity for a woman to heal, to strengthen herself, and to balance and harmonize her energies. The result of which is that she can live a long healthy life and make major contributions to her family, her community, and her life's mission. What mission you might say? I believe that each of us is born with a special mission that only we can accomplish. When we've completed our mission, it's time to leave. Part of your life's work is to discover what your mission is. There is something you were born to do. What is it? Deeply seated within you is the answer. TCM and especially Qigong can help you access this wonderful mystery. For many women, menopause can be the turning point, the time when they can finally touch their spirit in a meaningful way and discover their true power and deepest creativity.

Today, more than 95 percent of my patients are Western women. I find this most interesting, because I am not a Western medical doctor, but a doctor of traditional Chinese medicine, trained in the principles, theories, and technical practices of this ancient medicine. Yet, I find more and more women come to me because they are looking for a natural, effective way to relieve menopausal symptoms and a safe alternative to hormone replacement therapy. Some have been on estrogen replacement therapy (ERT) or HRT for years and are among the 20 percent who have experienced its side effects. Many have come to TCM as a last resort. I'm amazed when some of these women tell me that when they see their doctors, they will prescribe HRT immediately—automatically assuming that their patients will choose this path.

Today too, many of my patients come with menstrual or menopausal symptoms. Some are experiencing hot flashes, excessive bleeding, and night sweats, and a wide range of other health conditions that are familiar to women in the age range for menopause. Others, who are younger, come in search of ways to deal with PMS, cramps or migraine headaches, and perimenopause symptoms. Some are taking hormones, and others are looking for alternatives to them. I am happy to say that TCM can be of tremendous help to all these women.

THE ESSENTIAL DIFFERENCE OF TCM

As you get further into this book, you'll see that TCM works according to a completely different philosophy and system than Western medicine. While both can treat menopausal symptoms and reduce or eliminate a woman's suffering, the true result is not the same. During a woman's transition, TCM has the ability to help her adjust her body's Qi, or vital energy (something you will learn a lot about), in as little as a few months, or sometimes even weeks. This process may include acupuncture, Qigong, and ancient herbal formulas adapted for her specific needs. After her own healing ability has started to refunction, she does not have to come for acupuncture nor take Chinese herbs for the rest of her life.

With the proper support from TCM, she has just passed through this amazing gateway we've talked about. The patient who manages to reactivate her own healing ability has readjusted the balance of each of her major organs and restored harmony among them. She can now move on; unless she becomes ill or totally unbalances her major organ systems, she does not need to take anything else to remain healthy. The smartest women with the deepest insight about TCM return every two months to remain in balance and prevent problems. Why? Because TCM believes the best doctor is the one who prevents problems not treats them. We will talk more about working with a TCM doctor in Chapter 10.

Western medicine, on the other hand, has a different framework and tends to treat menopausal symptoms in isolation. And, because this framework does not have a deeper understanding or work with the source of the symptoms, the root causes are left unchanged and untreated. As you go through this book, you will gain important knowledge that you can apply immediately to your own health issues.

QI: THE SECRET BEHIND TCM

TCM always thinks about your health in terms of your Qi, or your life force. Its unique understanding of Qi is the true foundation of authentic TCM and is the basis of the efficacy of all its treatments, including acupuncture. TCM works from the premise that as long as your Qi remains strong and flows freely, and your body's organs work in harmony, disease or illness cannot enter—not even cancer! The opposite, however, is true as well. If your Qi is weak and not flowing freely, and your body's organs are not working in harmony, disease or illness can and do enter. You may be very surprised to learn about the ways in which TCM understands your body can be injured from what it considers internal and external pathogens.

Here's an analogy I like to use that I think most people can relate to. I tell my patients: "Think of your body as a car. Both your body and your car need power to run, but all the parts inside also have to function well. For your car to operate, it needs gas and a properly functioning engine. All the parts must be there; they must do what they're supposed to do. All the connections among the car's many parts must work too. Otherwise, even with plenty of gas, your car won't work well." It is virtually the same with the human body. You must have a certain level of Qi on which your whole body can depend to power itself for the tasks of your daily life. And, each organ, which has its own function, purpose, and Qi, must work in and of itself and then in harmony with your other organs or parts. Your body is an indivisible system within which every part has an affect on the other parts.

To understand the concept of Qi more deeply, it is important to note that TCM considers this invisible force as far more than just "pep," or stamina, or the kind of mental energy most of us in Western society run our lives on. Qi is the very life force of the Universe and the Qi of your body is connected to this force. Qi makes up the sun, the moon, the earth, and all things both living and nonliving. Everything has Qi and Qi gives everything life. Without it, there is no growth or change. Imagine a stagnant Universe with nothing flowing, growing, or moving! For us humans, it would be a place of unimaginable boredom and entropy. The important thing to understand about Qi is that, in all things, including the human body, Qi also carries information and a message. The strength of this message, and how far it carries, depends on the strength and quality of a person's Qi. A good TCM doctor knows all this and applies it in everything he or she does.

Understanding Qi is essential to menopause. When women with menopausal symptoms come to see me, virtually all of their problems are caused by a Qi imbalance. Generally speaking, this imbalance can be traced to the same source: kidney Qi deficiency and liver Qi stagnation. The kidney has become too weak to perform its regular functions and communicate its messages to its fellow organs; this condition is coupled with the problem of the liver's Qi being stuck in either an organ or a meridian. We will see how this double blow is the root cause of the many menopausal symptoms that Western women know so well.

My overall task as a TCM practitioner is not just to treat the condition of menopause. TCM treats the person and not the condition. So, it is critical to form a partnership with each patient within which she can spark her own healing power. This can help her through that special gateway where she can create the internal power to generate enough hormones for the rest of her life. How does TCM do this? Again, this approach differs from that of Western medicine. I like to tell my new patients: "I am not the bus driver. I do not make all the decisions. We must work together so that you can learn how to heal yourself. It is your body and you must take responsibility for healing yourself. My role is to help you and to motivate you and to offer you hope and strength." And, when we talk about healing, we talk about her body, mind, emotions, and spirit because TCM understands that they are inseparable and each affects the other. Together we work to boost her kidney Qi and help her liver function properly. This begins to bring her body back into balance and restore harmony to her organs. Together we also identify the things in her life that have caused these conditions to develop.

TCM has many tools from which to choose that have worked successfully for thousands of years for millions upon millions of Chinese women. There are foods for healing, ancient Chinese herbs and herbal formulas, acupuncture, moxibustion, and Tuina or acupressure, Qigong—and even Chinese psychology! This body of work is still in practice today.

In this book, I also want to pass on special ways you can heal yourself through particular foods that can be added to your daily diet. Most importantly, I want to share with you simple, but powerful Qigong movements called *Wu Ming* Meridian Therapy. These ancient self-healing movements, or meridian stretches, can increase your Qi, open up energy blockages, and prevent Qi stagnation. Practicing Qigong movements allows you to address the root cause of menopausal problems. They will help you build up your kidney Qi and relieve liver Qi stagnation. As with my own patients, we'll spend some time learning how each major organ is influenced by an emotion, and how an excess of that emotion can literally damage that organ's function. We will discuss what you can do to change your lifestyle and minimize stress, which can take a deadly toll on liver function.

DIFFERENCES IN APPROACH BETWEEN EAST AND WEST

As we've noted, Eastern and Western medicine approach menopause from two completely different points of view. In Western medicine, the main cause of menopausal symptoms is seen as a lack of estrogen production. Over the last hundred years or so, this natural transition has gradually been characterized as a "medical condition, or even disease." Consequently, the principal Western treatments prescribed for menopause have become drugs: ERT or HRT, which includes a form of progesterone in addition to estrogen. If we examine this approach a little closer, you can see that it raises some serious questions. Just because something is lacking doesn't necessarily mean that replacing it will restore normal function to a complex organism like the body. What has now become lacking—your hormone production—occurred as a result of a number of interrelated and interdependent physical, spiritual, and emotional changes.

We can understand this better by asking some simple questions. Think back to when you were younger. If you are pretty healthy today, why didn't you have a problem with hormone production then? What part of your body has caused this problem today? Is there a possibility that this condition can be fixed from the inside? Will HRT or ERT actually fix the real root problem? When? How long will it take to fix it? If you stop taking it, will the symptoms come back? If they do, how much longer must you take it to eliminate the problems? Infrequently is a Western woman given any useful knowledge about this natural biological transition and its holistic effect that surely involves her body, mind, and spirit—none of which can be separated, but must be treated as one whole system.

As you've seen, TCM sees menopause very differently. You've learned how TCM regards this transition as a time of natural decline in the body's kidney Qi. The treatment then involves helping a woman increase her overall Qi to make it strong and flowing, as well as helping to get her body's organs to work in harmony. If this can be achieved, TCM states that a woman can produce enough estrogen on her own for the rest of her life. I can assure you that many of my patients have faced a wide variety of menopausal issues and almost all of them have been helped successfully by TCM through this transition.

Let me explain how this works. TCM understands that estrogen production is related to the function of a healthy kidney (TCM uses the singular term "kidney" and "lung" to reflect its larger holistic understanding of these organs, including their physiological, spiritual, and emotional aspects as well). It also recognizes that estrogen is produced as a result of cooperation among several organs. The liver is an important partner in the production of estrogen. For your body to produce an adequate amount of this hormone, each of these organs must function properly by themselves, and, very importantly, they must also maintain harmonious communications with one another. The connections and the messages that flow back and forth between them are vital to maintain adequate estrogen production.

Let's look back to the time before your menopausal symptoms appeared. Certainly your body had enough estrogen then. So why is it missing estrogen today? According to TCM, it's because over a period of time, as your body ages, your Qi declines and your organs have lost their ability to work in harmony. When the messages between the organs become garbled, or unintelligible, or the power to transmit them weakens, your body begins to stop producing enough estrogen. According to TCM, this is the true root cause of all menopausal problems. And, when this condition is addressed and reversed, your body recaptures its natural ability to produce hormones. The level of hormone production will naturally be lower, but it will be enough to keep you healthy until your journey is over.

Think about the millions upon millions of women who have lived long lives without HRT. How did they do this? Surely not everyone of them suffered from debilitating symptoms. And, surely, it would not make sense, according to the natural law, to have an organism like the human body born without all the innate information and materials necessary for it to survive without outside drug intervention.

TREATING MENOPAUSE WITH TCM

TCM believes that the best cure is prevention. If you've reached menopause and have many uncomfortable symptoms, or are suffering greatly, your body has been out of balance for some time. Not everyone has a difficult transition; why is this happening to you? It's most likely that many warning signs appeared when you were younger, but you just didn't have the right information to decode them. I wish I could see more women when they're in perimenopause. If we could work together then, their menopause transition would very likely be a smooth and happy one.

If you take in hormones from the outside, your own power to produce them from within is diminished. These drugs can weaken the body's energy system. Your own Qi gets lazy, and the longer you take them, the less chance you have to heal yourself, and reactivate your ability to produce enough estrogen during your later years. On the other hand, if you take the opportunity to become balanced during menopause, you can reach a new level of health. And if you are healthy, you can heal yourself.

Here's an interesting way to look at how the body functions through the transition we call menopause. Suppose you have a well-running, healthy company that carries no debt whatsoever. All of its divisions are happy and prosperous. Internal communications among the various divisions is efficient, smooth, timely, and excellent. This is the equivalent of a healthy woman before she reaches menopause. Now, suppose this company is acquired in a merger. A new president is installed. The well-run company now has a change of leadership. Things are handled differently now and the internal divisions are, at worst, somewhat confused about how to proceed smoothly during this transition.

If your company enters this major transition in a healthy condition, it will have to make some adjustments for change, but it should experience very few problems. Because each division has been nurtured as a strong operating unit and, because communications among the divisions is still going smoothly, this transition should be a relatively easy one.

Suppose, however, that your company is carrying some financial debt; suppose your divisions are weak and perform erratically and that they have continually experienced internal problems. Suppose they are very territorial and dislike communicating with each other. In a company like this, any change will cause chaos. If a new president enters, then the company will definitely experience problems. This analogy helps illustrate what happens to many women during menopause. Where do you see yourself?

During menopause, if you take ERT or HRT, from the TCM standpoint, it's like going out and begging for a loan to keep your

company running. Now, your company's survival is based on outside assistance. The real question is how long can this go on without hurting the company as a whole? Without making your
company dependent on this outside source of aid? Wouldn't it be
better to fix the internal problems and regain balance and restore
harmony from within? In your body, the new president represents
your kidney (the main organ in charge of your estrogen production and overall Qi). Your other organs represent the internal divisions or systems that must continually communicate with each
other for maximum health.

What factors should you consider in making a choice
whether or not to go down a road less traveled by Western
women?

First of all, it's important to recognize that like you, no
women of menopausal age want to suffer from symptoms such as
hot flashes, night sweats, abnormal bleeding, emotional stress,
and more. Like you, many also worry about other age-related conditions such as heart disease, breast cancer, and osteoporosis. So
ERT and HRT, which are reported to reduce the risk of heart disease and slow bone loss and that are suggested by their physicians,
seem to provide a logical solution.

And why not? Heart disease is the number one cause of
death in the United States; it is responsible for half of all deaths
of women over age fifty. Osteoporosis is also a major health problem in this country; it afflicts more than 10 million Americans, 80
percent of whom are postmenopausal women. Osteoporosis
causes an estimated 1.5 million bone fractures annually, the most
damaging being hip fractures, which occur nearly seven times as
frequently in elderly women as in elderly men. Each year thousands of women die within several months of their fractures. The
survivors often end their days in nursing homes. These are grim
prospects indeed for women.

It is important to understand that hormonal therapy carries
many potential side effects and risks. It can also create new problems
in the course of solving old ones. For example, estrogen, which promotes cellular proliferation and growth, is a known tumor stimulant.

As such, if a woman chooses hormonal replacement, her trade-off is an increased risk of developing breast and/or uterine cancer.

According to the Cancer Statistical Review referenced in the Harvard Women's Health Watch, women who have been receiving HRT or ERT for five years or more have an overall 30 percent greater risk of breast cancer than those who have not. This translates into a real rise in risk from 10 percent to 13 percent. The following chart from the Cancer Statistical Review gives you an idea of the breakdown by age.

EFFECT OF HRT AND BREAST CANCER RISK

AGE	WITHOUT HRT	5 YEARS OF HRT
50–54	1 in 450	1 in 320
55–59	1 in 356	1 in 276
60–64	1 in 292	1 in 209
65–69	1 in 244	1 in 144

When used alone, as in ERT, estrogen has been shown to increase the risk of endometrial cancer (cancer of the lining of the uterus) by 400 to 800 percent. The risk of cancer increases with prolonged use of estrogen and with age. Ironically, in order to acquire whatever protection estrogen may offer from heart disease and osteoporosis, you must pass through the risk phase of breast cancer and keep taking these drugs.

To lower the risk of endometrial cancer, scientists developed another HRT composed of progestin (a synthetic form of the female hormone progesterone) and estrogen. Yet it, too, offers an imperfect solution (and has not been proven to reduce the risk of breast cancer). True, progestin allows the uterine lining to be shed, but it also promotes monthly bleeding for women undergoing HRT, as well as PMS and other menstrual symptoms.

From the TCM standpoint, continuing menstruation beyond its naturally occurring time span is not good. It literally forces a woman's body to go against the natural law. Losing blood every month long after this process should have ceased causes the body to waste a tremendous amount of its precious Qi. This is Qi, or life force, that can be conserved for longevity. Instead, it is diverted to support a situation that is not natural for the body's age.

TCM says that Qi and blood are inseparable; when you lose blood, you also lose Qi. When a woman is older, her body must work very hard and use up a lot of its Qi to replace menstrual blood. This also puts extra stress on the heart. Where does all this Qi or life force come from to make up more blood? Unfortunately, it is withdrawn from the kidney, your body's "energy savings account"—the very storehouse it depends on for longevity! So even if you're lucky enough to live into your seventies, eighties, nineties, and beyond, you will not be as strong and as healthy as you could have been. You have literally spent your inheritance and robbed yourself of the very life force or Qi you needed to protect your heart and bones.

I feel tremendous empathy for my Western patients. I see that they are caught between two fears: what might happen if they don't take hormones and what might happen if they do. In Western society, virtually all mainstream health authorities endorse only one treatment path. I do see some positive change in this direction, as some Western doctors shift their treatment to prescribing natural hormones and considering more natural approaches. Women who choose to avoid HRT are pretty much on their own and must figure out how to help themselves. Western women, for the most part, have no idea that there is another way—a time-tested way that can change their whole life. In China, these women would have great support from TCM. They would be able to go to any hospital or medical center in the country and be allowed to work with their doctors to choose between Eastern and Western medicine within the same institution.

Think about this. If many of America's most famous university medical centers or hospitals endorsed a way to treat menopause without hormones, which option would you chose? So many women go the route of HRT because they feel that they have no choice. More and more are actively searching for some natural way to manage their menopause. If you are on your own search, it is my hope that this book will show you that there is indeed another way—and a very powerful, very successful way at that. TCM can give women in Western society a natural and safe way out of this dilemma, one that can effectively treat the source and not the symptoms of menopause.

SHARING ANCIENT KNOWLEDGE

It is my privilege now to share with you what I have learned about TCM and menopause from my own masters, my own training and experiences, and from my exceptional patients who have decided to take the road less traveled. TCM is a medicine that is beyond the scientific and the measurable. As we've seen, its foundation stands rooted in the ancient understanding of Qi and our body as an inseparable energy system with its individual parts in constant communication with all other parts, and this whole amazing dynamic system wired, if you will, into the much larger one of the Universe. As we proceed through this information, I'd like you to remember that TCM is not a random collection of treatment options, single herbs, or visualization techniques. It is a complete healing modality whose principles and theories have existed unaltered for more than five thousand years. Above all, it understands how to see, really see, and treat the whole person—her body, mind, emotions, and spirit—each of which must be carefully nurtured for lasting health and longevity.

Little did I know when I first began studying TCM that my mission would become one of building bridges between the East and West for the ancient wisdom of this medicine. I believe, and so many of my patients believe, that the self-healing techniques of TCM can make a major contribution to women's health in Western society. My patients have taught me many, many things. Most importantly, they have shown me their desire and willingness to take responsibility for their own healing and to work for it. I am continually impressed by my patients' intelligence, sincerity, humor in the face of serious stress, and enthusiasm for finally connecting with something that makes sense to them. It is my wish that passing along this unique knowledge will help you and many more women transform themselves through the magnificent transition of menopause.

PART ONE

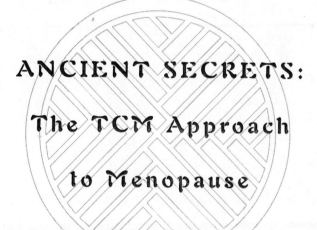

ANCIENT SECRETS:
The TCM Approach
to Menopause

To be a good doctor, you must understand that human health is related to environmental changes, seasonal changes, geographical effects, and changes in the Universal energies of yin and yang.

If you know all these things, you can really understand the physiological and pathological changes of the human body.

NEI JING (475-221 B.C.)

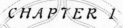

CHAPTER 1

TCM:
The Ancient Healing Practice
That Offers a Healthy Way Out of
Today's Hormone Dilemma

As you undoubtedly know from your own experience, menopause doesn't usually happen all at once. For most women, it comes on gradually over a period of years. No matter what stage you are in—from the early years (called perimenopause) when you body is preparing for the cessation of menstruation, through menopause, and after when your period has actually ended, TCM can support you and your health.

What characterizes these stages and their symptoms? During perimenopause, you may begin to experience such symptoms as irregular periods, mood swings, or frequent bouts of fatigue. If you've moved out of this prepatory state and progressed to menopause, then you may experience the much written about, full-blown menopausal symptoms of hot flashes, vaginal dryness, loss of sex drive, digestive and urinary problems, and more. If you are now in the postmenopause stage when your period has stopped, you may still have some lingering symptoms and you are now also more vulnerable to heart disease, breast cancer, and osteoporosis. At each of these stages, TCM provides a comprehensive framework for dealing with these and other symptoms, as well as a way to help you experience a healthy journey for the rest of your life.

Because many women are unfamiliar with TCM, the next logical questions, of course, are how does TCM work and how can it help me? To answer this fully, I'd like to take the time to provide some history about this ancient healing practice and its time-tested specialty of treating women's problems—particularly the diagnosis and treatment of menopause, or what TCM calls Menstrual Cycle Ending Symptoms.

TCM'S LONG HISTORY OF UNDERSTANDING A WOMAN'S BODY

TCM is alive and well today, practiced side-by-side with Western medicine in the top medical centers and hospitals of China. Just how old the healing art of TCM is no one really knows. Generally, it is considered among the most ancient in the world. It is the only one that has remained in continuous practice with a dedicated, government-supported system of practitioners, hospitals, colleges, and academies for more than five thousand years. Interest in TCM and its healing practices is growing rapidly worldwide. Today in the United States, there are more than sixty-five schools or institutes that teach acupuncture and Chinese herbal therapy.

The true origins of TCM occurred long before its principles and theories were written down twenty-five hundred years ago in the *Huang Di Nei Jing* (pronounced WHONG DEE NAY JEENG), considered to be the first TCM "textbook." This work is attributed to the Yellow Emperor, but scholars do not know who the real author is.

The *Huang Di Nei Jing* is a comprehensive work that outlines the entire structure of TCM and how it should be practiced. Among many things, it describes in sharp detail—without the aid of x-rays, computed tomography (CT) scans, or magnetic resonance imaging (MRIs)—the human body and how it works; the role of Qi and the meridians (energy pathways that carry Qi throughout the body and with which acupuncture is concerned);

as well as how the body interrelates with the spirit, the natural environment, and the greater Universe.

This remarkably comprehensive work addresses methods of diagnosis and treatment, as well as how to treat the source and not the symptoms of specific problems. It also describes the principle of prevention—the gateway to real health and longevity. This is especially relevant for women whose menopausal problems can be prevented well before they arrive at the transitional time in their lives. No other medicine has a specialty that has such a long-lived, practical, and practicable framework in prevention.

It is in this ancient text that we see the first references to women and their distinct life cycles. What the *Nei Jing* tells us is that a woman's Qi—and specifically her kidney Qi—moves in seven-year cycles. (A man's cycle is eight years long.) At the end of her first seven years, a healthy young girl's kidney Qi becomes abundant, manifesting itself in the growth of hair and permanent teeth. At fourteen years old, this Qi or life force, reaches its peak, causing the onset of puberty and the beginning of menstruation. A woman flourishes throughout her "fertile" years, and then at around age thirty-five, her Qi begins its natural decline. All men and women experience this natural energy decline (it's why and how we age), but how steeply and how rapidly your energy declines is actually under your control. This is a TCM concept that I think most Western women will be very interested in because so many of them really want to take responsibility for controlling their own health and healing. They are just looking for a healthy way to do it that works. Menopause usually occurs between the sixth and seventh cycles, or between the ages of forty-two and forty-nine. At this time, the *Nei Jing* tells us, a woman's kidney Qi begins to drop dramatically, menstruation ceases, and she may begin to experience many of the signs and symptoms of age.

The following chart indicates that, while kidney Qi declines normally over time, another course is possible. This other pathway can mean a delay in the onset of menopause and an increase in both the length and quality of a woman's life. This alternative

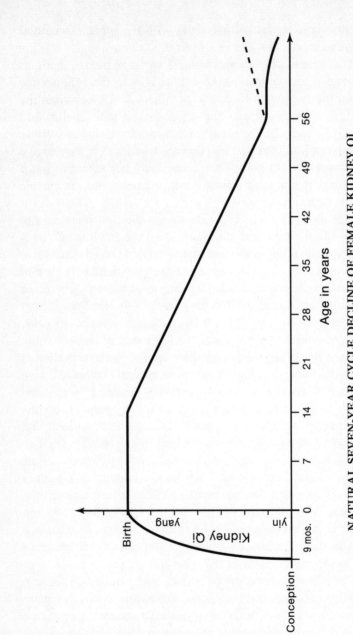

NATURAL SEVEN-YEAR CYCLE DECLINE OF FEMALE KIDNEY QI

course is only possible, however, if a woman takes care of herself so that she maintains her Qi at a higher level for a longer time.

When I think of this particular time in a woman's development, it reminds me of a warm fireplace where the fire has burned down to one small glowing ember that has almost disappeared. To get this fire going again, you must add wood and nurture that small single spark—not let it die. But it would be so much easier to rebuild this fire if it hadn't been left to dwindle down to just one tiny ember, wouldn't it? It's the same with your Qi. If you protect this life force and keep it safe and prevent internal and external factors from robbing its precious spark, you can stay well and live a long, healthy life, without constant medication and without serious illness. This concept is not something I invented yesterday so I could write this book; luckily it was firmly in place several thousand years ago and is a guiding principle of TCM. I always tell my patients, I am honored that you trust me, but you are really trusting in TCM!

OUR ENERGY SAVINGS AND CHECKING ACCOUNTS

The *Nei Jing* reveals a great deal about Qi. We learn from this early text that we have two different kinds of Qi—Inborn and Acquired. To better help my patients and you understand this concept, I've borrowed an almost ideal analogy from Western banking practices. I think almost everyone can relate to this explanation. I call Inborn Qi our savings account, and Acquired Qi our checking account.

Inborn Qi is the energy foundation that we inherit from our parents. This kind of Qi is stored in the kidney. Its quantity and quality are determined by the quantity and quality of your mother's and father's Qi; the kind of pregnancy your mother had; and the time, place, and nature of your birth. Your Qi or energy foundation cannot be changed. Most importantly, you have received a finite supply. It's like inheriting a piece of property. It can be rich or poor, filled with lush trees, or just a rocky patch. You have no control over the condition the gift is in. When my patients ask me, "How much Qi do I have?" I tell them it is up to fate. You do know deep inside, but this information is not readily available to you on a conscious level. I tell my patients TCM believes your life belongs to God, but your health belongs to you. These are the restrictions on your own unique energy legacy. Now, it's up to you. What you do with it, how you spend it, and how well you take care of it becomes your responsibility.

Ancient Chinese texts also tell us that Inborn Qi determines your basic constitution, both physical and mental, and governs your growth and development. If you have had children or had the opportunity to watch young children grow, you know what I am talking about. We often see that problems with Qi can be passed on to a child if, during a woman's pregnancy, her nutrition was poor or she was continually sick. For example, a baby born without strong Qi might have a soft spot on top of her head that closes later than normal; or a toddler might take longer to stand up because he or she doesn't have enough strength in the knees; or a child's dental development might be delayed. As you will see, each of these seemingly unrelated conditions can all be traced back to the workings of the kidney. A baby who is born prematurely will also have weak or deficient Qi and may experience some of the symptoms I've just described.

All of the above problems are related to the bone; in TCM, all matters related to the bone are controlled by the kidney—the storehouse of Inborn Qi. In working with babies and children who have bone problems, I always treat their kidney with an herb tonic or bone soup to strengthen this organ. Bone soup can be made from any kind of bones with marrow (you'll find a recipe in Chapter 15). Problems of Inborn Qi (and therefore kidney problems) in young children can show up in other ways too. Among them might be bed-wetting or delayed menses.

TCM says that the quantity and quality of our Inborn Qi also determines how long we live. Even though TCM believes this is true, it also recognizes that how we manage our allotted time is up to each of us. TCM believe that everyone has a mission. The nature of your mission may not be readily accessible to you, but when your mission is accomplished, it's time to leave this earth plane. Unfortunately for many of us, we rely far too heavily on our savings account of Inborn Qi; we use its precious "funds" wastefully. When we've emptied this account, it's literally time to die.

Luckily, the *Nei Jing* describes another readily available source from which we can withdraw energy—Acquired Qi, or our checking account. Acquired Qi supports the function of all the organs, and helps maintain the body's ability to regulate and heal itself. The good part about this checking account of Acquired Qi is that (unlike our savings account), we can actually make daily deposits of Qi to it. How? By eating high-quality foods in the proper amounts at the proper times; by ensuring that our organs are functioning well and in harmony; by practicing energy-conserving Qigong movements; and by learning how to manage our Qi. Thus, our personal checking account is dynamic and allows Qi to constantly flow in and move out. By generating and managing Acquired Qi, we have a daily chance to maximize the power and harmonious functioning of our own body's system.

Unfortunately, most people don't build up enough Acquired Qi in their checking accounts and must routinely withdraw "funds" from their savings accounts of Inborn Qi for the day-to-day energy expenditures of life's activities. These include respiration, metabolism, healing from internal and external assaults, sleeping, eating, digestion, elimination, thinking, feeling, intuition, and more! This is particularly true for modern women who are constantly on the go as professional professionals: professional mothers, professional volunteers, with many more roles. As a result, when many Western women reach menopausal age, their Inborn Qi—their savings account stored in the kidney—is often depleted. They may not know this, but they can feel it and experience it in the many symptoms we're about to discuss. This problem is compounded by the fact that stressful lifestyles also take a major toll on liver function.

As a result, women are experiencing menopause earlier, have greater and more frequent symptoms, and are being diagnosed with breast cancer and osteoporosis in greater numbers than ever before.

These linked checking and savings accounts are a lifetime package deal. TCM understands that the human body does not work in any other way. Their operating rules are related to natural, not man-made, law; they are very strict and cannot be changed. You can begin to appreciate why it's so important to build up your checking account continuously and be extremely cautious about the irreplaceable Qi in your savings account. One ancient Chinese doctor described this relationship a different way: "Your life is like a candle—you can be born with a small one, or a tall one. You have no choice in this. How to protect its flame is now up to you. If you've been given a long candle and you burn it carelessly, you will not last as long as a shorter candle that protects its flame. The better you protect your light the longer it remains lit."

AS TCM GROWS, SO DOES ITS UNDERSTANDING OF WOMEN'S PROBLEMS

Over time, the body of TCM's healing knowledge expanded, and women's health issues became one of TCM's specialties. By A.D. 610, one of the most comprehensive TCM textbooks on women's health was compiled by a number of practitioners. It describes more than two hundred thirty-eight different conditions and divides them into two main categories: obstetrics and gynecology. This medical work also outlines special herbal formulas to address most of these conditions. While the words defining these specialties were not used at that time, the types of care were explicitly clear. This specialty continued to develop and in A.D. 852 the earliest TCM medical textbook devoted exclusively to pregnancy was written. Much of this information and many of its formulas are still used to this day.

Throughout the ages, Chinese doctors developed a wide range of healing practices to treat women. In addition to providing information about treatment options, ancient texts also describe in great detail the relationship between practitioner and patient, and specifically the roles that both must play in the healing process.

TCM looks at medicine as an art, and the source behind that art is, of course, Qi. Therefore, those who practice this medicine are considered to be like any real artist. You are either born with this "gift" or not. A good TCM doctor knows this is true. Therefore, he or she regards the various healing methods as vehicles to transfer his or her gift of healing to the person who is unbalanced physically or ill. To do so, TCM texts say, it is a matter of profound communication between practitioner and patient. It is the doctor's task to choose the best treatment designed specifically for that individual. Likewise, it is the patient's responsibility to be an open and willing recipient of care. If this mutually respectful relationship is not in place, it is difficult to achieve the best results.

In ancient times, there were many famous doctors who would not work with patients who did not believe in the treatment. A good TCM practitioner understands that you must treat the whole person and not just her disease. Because of this, the TCM practitioner can also save Qi by connecting with the patient's own and helping her jump start it; otherwise, the practitioner needs to spend his or her own healing Qi to help the patient.

Even if the patient is not well, as long as her healing ability hasn't been damaged beyond repair, her body's Qi and its energy field is ten times more powerful than the doctor's. Think about your car when it has a dead battery. If your battery is in good condition, once your car receives a jump start and the engine begins to run, you can continue on your own. If your battery needs to be replaced, then the car has to be towed, which take a lot more energy, time, and cost. Like your car battery, if your own Qi can be sparked, then your body will do the job of healing. If, for some reason, my patient doesn't believe in her treatment, I have to fix her problem without the benefit of cooperation. I have to do the whole job and consequently spend a lot more of my own Qi in the process. We also may have to spend more time. Even if we manage to achieve some success, the problem can return, because the patient hasn't used her own healing power to help fix herself.

Here's one way to look at this concept: There are two ways I can help you with your math homework. I can simply give you the answers; or, I can show you where to go and how to get the answers. If I help you learn how to get the answers, you will be able to pass your math test, and you will be able to go beyond this one test and apply your knowledge again and again. Or, it's like baking, I can buy you a cake with nice frosting, or I can show you how to make your own. When you can make your own, you will not need my help any more. You can do it yourself, and you can do it whenever you want to. My goal as a TCM practitioner is to really help you heal yourself and learn how to tap your own healing ability. I like to make a joke with my patients. I tell them: "From the business perspective, I should want to see you as many times as possible. From the TCM perspective, I should want to get you out of my office as quickly as possible."

By believing and thereby cooperating, TCM understands that you can accomplish two very important things: you can actually trigger something inside you that allows your healing ability to reawaken and function, and your healing ability can amplify the doctor's help.

It's important for me to repeat again that all TCM healing methods are tools designed to strengthen or increase an individual's Qi through a deep communications process. Ironically, TCM believes that it doesn't really matter which technique practitioners use. Think about it this way: I can communicate with you through e-mail, fax, a personal letter, or by telephone. Each has its advantage, but in the long run, it doesn't really matter which method I choose. I am getting a message to you. It's the same with TCM's tools. They all have the same goal: to communicate the healing message through the transfer of Qi.

Different TCM healing methods have their advantages. Some work from the outside in (e.g., acupuncture) and others work from the inside out (herbs). Some act more quickly and others are more slow and deliberate. Some work well with other treatments;

some work best alone. It is the task of a TCM practitioner to use whatever he or she can to maximize the benefit for the improvement of the whole person.

In general, I find that acupuncture can help improve and strengthen your body's overall function. It's like a major tune-up for your whole body. From my experience and knowledge, for example, it is one of the best ways to help the liver function better because it stimulates the meridian channels. Acupuncture is particularly good for relieving stagnation of Qi or blood, and to help promote the flow of Qi. On the other hand, I find that classical herbs are best for the kidney and the lung. They are good for increasing Qi or blood. They are also effective in addressing an organ or meridian deficiency or an organ function disorder. Again, each treatment has its unique purpose, and a good TCM doctor should know when and how to apply this knowledge in a practical way. However, the combination of disease and today's fast-paced lifestyle have presented TCM practitioners with an enormous challenge. In my own practice, I find I have to use a variety of methods, and an innovative combination of methods, to help Western women heal.

This is not surprising because today's lifestyles are so vastly different from the much more simple ancient Chinese lifestyles when these healing methods were revealed many centuries ago. This also goes directly to the heart of how TCM must be practiced. It is a medicine of individuality and one of its treatment principle states that you must be treated according to: who you are, where you are, when you are, and how you are. We will look at treatment principles in depth in Chapter 10. You can easily see, though, that TCM finds it essential to treat you as you because you are unique. When I treat my menopausal patients, I cannot simply ignore the fact that they are Western women; that their diets are different, that their stress levels are different, and that they have grown up on a different land mass than their Chinese counterparts. It will become very clear to you that TCM is definitely not a "one size fits all" medicine, though there are certain things that work to some degree for virtually all patients, like *Wu*

Ming Meridian Therapy, because we are all under the same natural law, and virtually everyone needs to increase Qi.

THE HEALING TOOLS

The earliest written works about different healing methods appeared around the third century A.D. Up until that time, TCM had been an oral tradition passed down secretly by practitioners from generation to generation. Even before the recent Communist rule, Chinese culture had long been a secret society. Until recently, it was not a common practice to share our healing traditions and what we know with the outside world. That is one reason why it has taken so long for TCM to reach the hearts and minds of Westerners. The airing of Bill Moyer's *Healing and the Mind* television series on the Public Broadcasting System was one major step forward in making a wide audience aware of the power of TCM and Qigong.

It is time to introduce TCM even more broadly. This, I believe, is part of my mission and certainly something I can do in gratitude for the many gifts TCM and my masters have given me. Here are TCM's most important healing tools that we will discuss in relation to menopause.

Qigong

Sometime in the A.D. mid-200s, the illustrious TCM practitioner, Dr. Hua Tuo, became the first Chinese doctor not only to perform orthopedic surgery, but also to understand the need for Qi to move through the body to accelerate recovery. He created a powerful series of Qigong (CHEE KUNG) movements, which are movements for self-healing to do just that. Dr. Tuo adapted them from observing the movements of various animals. Today in parks all over China, you can still see hundreds of thousands people practicing this popular form of Qigong known as Wu Qin Xi (OOH SHING CHEE).

I call Qigong a "practice." TCM has understood its efficacy for millennia as one of the most remarkable and powerful energy enhancers available to us. We know it can greatly benefit women of all ages, with or without menopausal symptoms. Qigong is actually the most important healing tool I can share with you. It is something you can do easily each and every day not only to heal yourself, but also to add Qi to your energy checking account! I explain Qigong in general in Chapter 10, and specific self-healing energy movements called *Wu Ming* Meridian Therapy for menopausal symptoms in Chapter 14. This information has never before been shared with a Western audience. When you begin practicing, you should understand that this is a healing gift that will last a lifetime. Qigong can be done anywhere, anytime, by just about anyone, and without any special equipment.

I want you to know that I too "practice" every spare moment I have. Because I am a healing practitioner, I'm always giving away Qi. So it's vital for me to generate my Acquired Qi through this discipline.

Acupuncture and Moxibustion

Around the same time Qigong was being described, another ancient healing art was documented for posterity. It is the classical work on acupuncture written by Huang Fumi more than eighteen hundred years ago. In his remarkable text, he identified the 349 acupoint locations on the body, their therapeutic properties and contraindications, as well as methods of needle manipulation. This information is still used today by Chinese doctors and acupuncturists. Huang Fumi also provided us with information about moxibustion, the application of heat to acupoints to heal certain conditions.

Acupuncture is the healing method that has most captured the minds and imagination of Westerners. The word actually has Latin roots, where "acus" means needle and "puncture" means to rupture or make a hole. So acupuncture means to puncture with a needle. The Chinese word for it is *Zhen*. Although we'll talk about this practice in a deeper way in Chapter 10, here we can say that TCM uses this technique to disperse blocked Qi in the meridian channels or passageways by inserting needles into key points along these energy routes. Acupressure uses deep massage to stimulate these same key points. Moxibustion uses heat instead of needles on specific acupoints to stimulate the flow of Qi. Each treatment technique is unique and is used by TCM for different health conditions. Skilled and well-trained TCM practitioners know when and how to use these healing techniques to achieve the best healing results.

CLASSICAL CHINESE HERBS

Around the same time that Huang Fumi was writing about acupuncture, the most important texts about Chinese herbs were also being written down. One book has more than 262 prescriptions for the treatment of diseases at varying stages. From this classical text, TCM practitioners learn that even different stages require different kinds of herbs. This particular body of work laid the foundation for herbal prescriptions that are taught to this day in TCM colleges and hospitals.

Another book, translated as *The Herbal*, was written during the fourth century A.D. It summarized the then-known Chinese pharmaceutical knowledge, detailing more than 365 kinds of drugs and pharmacological theories. Interestingly, many of these have proven extremely valuable to modern clinical practice. For example, it recommends a very simple formula to help treat mood swings experienced by some menopausal women that is still used very successfully today. All you do is eat a mixture of boiled Chinese dates, wheat, and licorice. (For more information about recipes for menopausal conditions read Chapter 15.)

It's important to note that these early doctors of TCM understood the properties of herbal substances in a much deeper context than the scientific. This recognition of and working with the Qi or energy properties of herbs is what makes TCM herbal prescriptions work so effectively. In other words, these ancient doctors had the extraordinary insight and sensitivity to understand which herbs could enter specific meridians or organs for healing purposes. They also showed us how to use the herbs to re-create a better environment in the body so that it can jump start its own healing capabilities. As we've noted, your body is ten times smarter and ten times more powerful than you think, but at times (especially when we're ill and out of balance), it takes a good doctor of Chinese medicine to put it back on track.

According to these classical texts, herbs should be prepared using a special formula that people of the West might call a prescription. An herbal remedy can be a single, very powerful formula, or it can be a combination of three or four herbs that are aimed at relieving the acute symptoms as well as going deeper to address the root cause.

Remarkably, all this medical documentation took place a very long time ago—around the time the Roman Empire was collapsing!

TCM PSYCHOLOGY

A number of other treatment theories evolved through the centuries, including the specific times of the day and seasons that are best for treatment. Beginning with the *Nei Jing*, there are also thousands of pages and many texts concerning Chinese psychology. Dr. Zhang (A.D. 1156-1228) was the first doctor to create a medical text outlining his work using psychology to treat various problems. These ancient case studies illustrate how to use emotions to treat physical problems that have their root cause in excess emotions. TCM has a framework for treating emotion-based illnesses. It says that if the problem is caused by something emotional, then something emotional must be used to address the root cause. Without understanding the source of a condition, it is almost impossible to treat it effectively. And, often there is the potential to do some very real harm. I think you'll find the story about women who seek relief from sinus problems in Chapter 5 very interesting in light of this concept. It's also interesting to note that Dr. Zhang's work predates the work of Dr. Sigmund Freud, considered the father of Western psychiatry, by more than seven hundred years.

FOODS

TCM believes that food is a very powerful medicine and understands its value in preventing or treating a problem. Unlike today's thinking about food as a healing resource that concentrates on its physical properties, TCM understands food from the unique perspective of Qi or healing energy. My patients find it extremely beneficial to learn how to make adjustments in their daily food choices to complement other forms of treatment.

TCM'S CONTRIBUTION TO WORLD MEDICINE

Today TCM is flourishing in China. It is used effectively with Western medicine to treat a variety of diseases and illnesses. In a number of instances, TCM offers a significant advantage over Western medicine—especially in the treatment of chronic conditions or sports injuries. Frequently, TCM can also help individuals with certain health problems that Western medicine can no longer treat. For some, the results can seem like a miracle.

Today, if you go to a TCM hospital in China (as many do), you will find that TCM is divided into eleven departments or specialties. These specialties have existed for more than six hundred years. They are: general internal problems, orthopedics, skin problems, gynecology, pediatrics, ophthalmology; ear, nose, and throat; acupuncture, Tuina or acupressure, Qigong, and hemorrhoids (most people don't know that TCM specializes in the treatment of hemorrhoids).

A nationwide study done a decade ago in China found that there were more than forty thousand practitioners, fifteen hundred hospitals with more than one hundred thousand beds, twenty-six colleges, and thirty academies of TCM. In a recent meeting with Zonghan Zhu, M.D., of the Beijing Municipal Health Bureau and the World Health Organization (WHO) Collaborating Center for Epidemiology, I learned that 15 million permanent and temporary residents of Beijing are now being served by an increasing number of TCM hospitals. Dr. Zhu said that, within the past ten years, eighteen TCM hospitals had been built at both the municipal and district or county level to better serve Beijing's population. He also told me that even general hospitals in China are required to set up a separate department of TCM and a separate pharmacy devoted to TCM classical formulas and herbs.

Despite the fact that TCM has been around for a very, very long time, the general public worldwide is only now becoming familiar with its practice. Over the years, however, the scientific community has recognized Chinese medicine's early and valuable discoveries and their contributions to the world's medical knowledge. For instance, TCM is credited with identifying food and water as sources of parasitic infections. By the eleventh century A.D., the Chinese had already made enormous strides in immunology, specifically in the treatment of smallpox—that's nine hundred years before the vaccine was "discovered" by Edward Jenner in 1796. In fact, TCM texts refer to Chinese doctors inoculating people with smallpox material through the nostrils as early as 600 B.C.! Doctors of TCM also correctly identified how disease is spread through the air and helped develop some of the earliest theories of epidemiology. Until this information was written, it was believed that all illness or diseases could only enter the body through its surface.

And now today, more and more, TCM is finding its way to a much broader and highly interested general public and individuals such as yourself who believe they can benefit from this unique body of healing wisdom. Over the past few years, my Center has done a great deal of work to help educate Western audiences about TCM. We've held numerous workshops at the Center and in cooperation with other Centers and hospitals throughout the New York metropolitan area. For close to three years I also contributed the first-ever column on TCM to a national consumer health magazine. I am also pleased to say that our foundation has launched the first nationally distributed newspaper dedicated to educating Western consumers and health care professionals about TCM. It is called *Traditional Chinese Medicine World*. Besides having a large practice that helps women with menopausal symptoms, I also have special healing programs for women with breast cancer. Our Website at www.breastcancer.com now receives more than 1.5 million accesses per year.

In the United States today, there is a national board—the National Commission for Certification of Acupuncture and Oriental Medicine (NCCAOM)—that certifies approximately 700 to one thousand new acupuncturists through a comprehensive examination given twice a year. (There are about thirteen thousand practicing acupuncturists nationwide.) The NCCAOM's certifying standards are used by thirty-five states and Washington, D.C. Three states—California, Louisiana, and Nevada—have their own. Furthermore, another organization, the Council of Colleges of Acupuncture and Oriental Medicine, currently has more than thirty-nine colleges of acupuncture, TCM, and oriental medicine who have been through, or are in the process of, an accreditation effort. And most important, in 1998 the National Institutes of Health (NIH) recognized and approved the use of needle acupuncture for certain health conditions including pain relief. Two years prior to that the U.S. Food and Drug Administration (FDA) reclassified acupuncture needles from experimental medical devices to the same regulated category as surgical scalpels and hypodermic syringes.

With the quantum leap in the ability to communicate information worldwide at speeds undreamed of in the past, the door to traditional Chinese medicine is now swinging open for many more people. In the March 1998 edition of the *Harvard Health Letter*, the FDA estimates that Americans are now spending about $500 million a year on acupuncture treatments. They are also making between nine to twelve million visits to practitioners yearly.

While this increasing interest is exciting, I must caution you about the importance of learning how to identify a skilled TCM practitioner, how to work effectively with him or her, and how to recognize a true healer, if you are lucky enough to meet one. One of my masters taught me the nature of a very high level healer with this simple advice. "To become a true healer," he said, "you must carry your head and treat your patients." When I asked him what this meant, he went on: "You must put your life . . . you must put your ego . . . you must put your fame . . . you must put everything behind you and only care about the life of your patient." It is often difficult to know how to find a good TCM practitioner. Intuition plays a major role. After you read this book, I think you will be able to find the right TCM doctor for you.

Most of all, it is my hope that you will take away from this book a much more in-depth understanding of TCM and a deeper appreciation for its principles, theories, and treatments. Whether you are entering perimenopause, going through menopause, or have reached the other side of menopause, I know that the ancient wisdom in this book can take you through this special transition without hormones. You will now have the knowledge to reawaken your own healing ability and take advantage of life's final opportunity to strengthen yourself for the journey ahead. Remember that no matter what, this healing power is always within you.

TO SUMMARIZE:

- TCM has been in continuous practice with a government-supervised system of colleges and academies, hospitals, and practitioners for more than five thousand years.
- TCM's principles and theories were first written down in a landmark medical cannon called the *Huang Di Nei Jing*, written more than twenty-five hundred years ago. This work is commonly attributed to the Yellow Emperor.
- The *Nei Jing* details how the human body looks and works; the role of Qi and meridians; diagnoses and treatment methods; and provides important knowledge about women and their life cycle.
- According to the *Nei Jing*, a woman's Qi, specifically her kidney Qi, moves in seven-year cycles. By the age of thirty-five, Qi begins to decline naturally

and drops dramatically between the ages of forty-two and forty-nine. As a result, menstruation ceases and many signs and symptoms of aging may appear.

- Our bodies have two different kinds of Qi: Inborn and Acquired. I refer to them as energy "savings" and "checking" accounts, respectively.

- Inborn Qi is the life force we inherit from our parents. It cannot be changed or replenished.

- Acquired Qi is life force we produce from food, energy movements, and healing treatments, and positive lifestyle habits that allow us to consciously manage our Qi.

- TCM is considered an art form. Accordingly, true healers are like true artists or musicians, they are born not taught. They possess the intuition and the insight to go beyond the tools and techniques of the system.

- TCM believes that its healing methods are tools that can be applied to help the individual strengthen or increase Qi through a deep communication process between practitioner and patient.

- TCM's main healing tools are food, Qigong, acupuncture, Tuina or acupressure, moxibustion, herbal therapy, and psychology.

- Although TCM has not been well known in Western cultures, its practitioners are recognized as significant contributors to world medicine in areas such as immunology, epidemiology, herbal therapy, and more.

- Today, interest in TCM is growing rapidly and is becoming more accessible to people in the West.

CHAPTER 2

Seven Steps to Self-Healing with TCM for a Hormone-Free Menopause

I have developed a seven-step guide to self-healing with TCM for menopause. The number seven is significant because it has an important relationship with the lifetime energy cycles through which a woman lives. TCM believes that women's cycles are seven years long, while men's are eight.

According to TCM theory, every seven years marks a distinct cycle of life changes for females. After two cycles, around the age of fourteen when many young girls begin to menstruate, their Qi or life force begins to decline with each new seven-year cycle. After seven cycles, around the age of forty-nine, a woman's Qi reaches its lowest point. If I can help a woman rebalance her Qi and reignite her life force (remember the yang Qi and the ember in the fireplace?) before it fades out completely, then a woman can actually return to the healthy state of her earlier years. This reflects one of nature's energy laws, which we see in the normal cycle of the year's seasons.

You can see this cyclical flow in the diagram that the Chinese call the BaGua with its Twelve Energy Messages Chart on page 24. Let's look at how this BaGua configuration reflects the natural cycle of a whole year's Qi, as well as the natural cycle of your lifetime's Qi or life force.

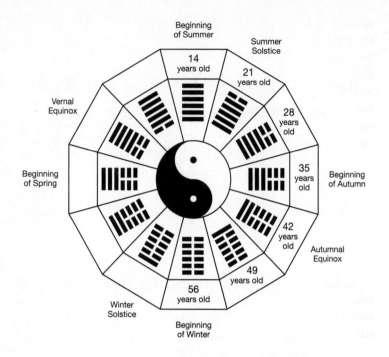

THE BAGUA ENERGY CHART

In the BaGua diagram above, solid lines represent yang Qi, while broken lines represent yin Qi. At the top of the chart, you can see that there are six solid lines; these represent the highest time of yang Qi, or kidney Qi. For a woman, it also represents the time before her first menstrual cycle. As we follow the segments around the BaGua, you can see that every seven years, the lines at the top become progressively broken until the six solid lines become six broken lines. This point, which marks a woman's fifty-sixth year, represents the state of lowest yang Qi.

Now, notice in the next segment, that the lines begin to become solid again. As we follow the BaGua's natural progression of these segments around to the top, they continue their flow until all the lines become solid again. And so it goes; this is nature's endless cycle. Because TCM theories state that we are part of nature, it should be possible to follow this flow within our own bodies. However, to reach this kind of union and match our own Qi with nature's own Qi, there are many requirements that need to be met to make the body, mind, and spirit work as a complete unit. In today's high-stress world, it is almost impossible to recharge oneself at the moment of the lowest yang Qi, but in theory it is possible to round this curve and rejuvenate one's self. Although we may never see them in the news, I believe that there are special people today who are able to do this.

SEVEN SELF-HEALING STEPS THAT CAN REGENERATE YOUR LIFE FORCE AND HELP YOU MAKE A MAGNIFICENT TRANSITION THROUGH MENOPAUSE

1. Discover your own healing power by learning how your body really works. Become familiar with the principles and theories of TCM. Learn how to generate Qi, conserve Qi, and how to use Qi wisely.

2. Take inventory. Answer the questions on the self-healing TCM checklists in Chapter 11 and test your knowledge about what can really heal or harm your body. See how they apply to your current state of health or how they relate to the menopausal symptoms you may be experiencing. Use the answers as a guide to identify areas of your life where you can change behavior to conserve and strengthen your kidney Qi and relieve liver stagnation. Remember, for Western women, these are the two root causes of menopausal symptoms. You can do a lot to heal yourself by studying these checklists.

3. Create a calm, peaceful, positive lifestyle that can help your body make the transition through menopause more easily.

4. Discover how your mental powers can create dramatic change from the inside out. Learn the classical secrets and true shortcuts to achieving a long, healthy life.

5. Learn the eight ancient Qigong movements that can help you recall your own natural healing power. Practice *Wu Ming*

Meridian Therapy for twenty minutes at least once a day. You will be amazed at the cumulative benefits.

6. Use the healing power of foods and herbs to support your body through this life change. Create your own unique "Eating for Healing Plan" with the foods in Chapter 15. Study the classical herbs and healing recipes with herbs in this chapter. Incorporate as many as possible into your daily plan.

7. Discover how to use nature's own Qi to support your healing journey. Remember going against nature's law can create illness and waste precious Qi. So, pay attention to nature's changes.

I'd like to remind you that, for most women, menopause is not an event, but a process. It's something that happens gradually over time. Therefore, the ability to avoid or eliminate menopausal symptoms should be viewed from the process perspective as well. The seven steps outlined above make up a self-healing blueprint that you can begin to work with at any age; however, the earlier you begin the stronger you can become. And, I mean strong in a holistic way, especially in your own spirit.

Many Western women believe they are taking reasonably good care of themselves. Very often, they are surprised by what I tell them they should do to become really well. To give you an idea of how a woman who believes that she is doing everything possible to stay healthy, finds herself suffering from a broad range of menopausal symptoms, let's follow the story of Jane. "Jane" is a composite patient who represents so many of the Western women who come to me for help. I am deeply moved by their predicaments and I hope by telling this story you will gain a better insight into your own health issues and begin to understand the importance of this seven-step TCM self-healing guide. I hope you will use this knowledge to help other women as well.

COMPOSITE PATIENT

We first look in on Jane when she's a young girl. She's a typical American girl who has started menstruating at the age of fourteen years. She's fun and inquisitive, enjoys soccer, does well in school (although tests stress her out), has a pretty happy home life, and loves to eat out at fast food restaurants. In her last year in high school, Jane is accepted into a local college where she is also given a work scholarship. In her junior year of college, she begins to develop cramps every once in a while when her period comes. Occasionally, she will also develop headaches, but they go away when she takes painkillers. And, she also notices that every month her skin breaks out. Jane hopes to go on to graduate school, so she studies for her classes, fulfills her responsibilities for the work scholarship, and occasionally moonlights at various campus jobs to save extra money for her advanced degree.

If Jane were to see a TCM doctor at this stage of her life, she might be surprised at the amount of time and attention the TCM practitioner would give to her cramps, headaches, and skin problems. According to TCM, these are early warning signals that the function of the organs related to the menstrual cycle is out of balance. If she is not helped to rebalance this condition, she could be heading for a more serious event that TCM calls a liver function disorder.

Her TCM doctor would ask her about what is going on in her life and why her Qi is becoming out of balance at such a young age. They would discuss the increasing stress she's under and the current demands of her college life. The TCM doctor would work with her to prescribe certain herbs to help rebalance her Qi. He would also recommend that she take it easy, let her anger and frustration go, and help Jane identify ways that her stress can be relieved.

If he's a wise TCM practitioner, he will also encourage her to look ahead a few decades and realize that what she does at this time in her life will have profound consequences on her health and the way she will feel when she reaches her forties, fifties, and beyond. For Jane, a child of Western culture, it would be a big stretch to think that many years ahead, especially when it comes to her health. At this point in her life, these intermittent problems would only be regarded as an annoyance or an inconvenience. Even if she went to a Western doctor with her headaches, cramps, and skin problems, her scientific tests would most likely be normal. And as empathetic and concerned as her doctor would be, she would most likely have to send Jane to several different doctors to evaluate each of her problems. Because of its framework for understanding the whole body, her TCM doctor would relate all three conditions to one organ and meridian that is out of balance or harmony, the liver. Jane wants to stay well and at this point in her life reads lots of books and magazines about how to do this. Her TCM doctor would advise her to slow down, relieve the stress in her life, and ask her to stop eating so many cold foods and drinking so many cold beverages, which, as you will learn, play a role in the root cause of certain serious health conditions.

Change, however, is very difficult for Jane. All her teen and young adult life, she has been inundated with messages that she has come to accept as true. There is no way for her to know that there are other paths and other thoughts about how to remain truly healthy. Not too many of her favorite magazines, TV shows, or books, have ever told her that she was born with the power to heal herself—not just from the garden variety of sniffles, coughs, colds, scrapes and cuts, and indigestion, but from real health problems.

Let's look in on Jane again after she's finished graduate school and has taken her first job. She is very eager to please her bosses. And because she is smart and competent, she is given more and more responsibility, which comes with increasing levels of stress. Jane is young and believes she can handle the stress. She also has no idea of its real impact on the healthy function of her liver. Like so many young people, she takes for granted her stamina, her good health, and her ability to endure long hours at work and late nights out with her friends. Soon, Jane falls in love. Having dated a number of men, Jane believes this is the person for her, but after two and a half years of building a relationship, things simply don't work out. She breaks up with her boyfriend, and is deeply affected by this event. There are now a number of emotional upheavals that follow in her life. Jane notices that when her emotions are out of balance, her headaches, cramps, and skin problems worsen. Still, she has no framework for connecting them with one root cause.

A friend refers Jane to a TCM practitioner who is an acupuncturist and herbalist. She visits the TCM doctor because her menstrual cycle has stopped for a few months; she now has a vaginal discharge. Sleep disturbances are beginning to cause day-time fatigue. She still has skin problems and they're getting worse. Also, she has developed constipation and breast tenderness. The doctor tells Jane how critical it is to address her condition of liver Qi stagnation. After several acupuncture treatments, Jane's period returns. She makes some dietary changes, her broken heart mends, and her emotions become stable again. Jane is determined to take good care of herself and starts to learn how to meditate. For about a decade, she remains in relatively good health.

During this time, Jane marries. She is unaware of it, but she has managed to transform herself somewhat so her energy vibration is different than when she was younger. Inevitably, because she has changed, everyone around her changes to some degree. Some changes are for the better, others for the worse.

In time, Jane becomes pregnant. She works during her pregnancy because it helps ease her family's financial concerns. Without much rest, or much thought about what she might need to heal herself from the physical, emotional, and mental changes of pregnancy and childbirth, Jane returns to work almost immediately after her child—a beautiful, active baby girl—is born.

Again, because she is good at her job, Jane is given more responsibilities. Between her heavy work schedule and her family obligations, she actually forgets to take care of herself. There just doesn't seem to be time for anything in her life. Jane tells herself that it won't always be like this. Over time, she has had to put off her yoga and meditation classes. Her diet has taken a turn for the worse. Almost always, she works through her lunchtime, eating, answering her e-mail, and making phone calls at the same time. Almost always she eats cold foods and drinks cold diet sodas. At this point, Jane has begun to develop frequent headaches across the front of her head and a nagging back pain that stays with her pretty much most of the time.

About three years later, Jane has her second child. Although she loves her husband and her two children deeply, she feels anxious when she's not at work. She feels anxious when she's at work and not at home with her family also. Although she had planned to stay at home for a longer time with her second child, Jane changes her plans and returns to her job within a few months. Naturally, the rest she really needed to recover from her second pregnancy and childbirth never happens.

Two years later, her energy seems to be a lot lower than it used to be. Once in a while she sees a chiropractor to relieve her back pain. Occasionally, she'll revisit her acupuncturist who always gently reminds her that she did not take care of a number of problems that arose after childbirth, and that she should work at healing them now so that she doesn't encounter problems later with menopause. But, Jane can only find the time to come once in awhile; when she feels better she stops. She really believes she's trying to protect her own health. She can only do a little bit and unfortunately, it's never enough.

One Christmas, both sets of parents come for an extended visit. Jane catches a simple cold. Not wanting to put a damper on all the festivities planned, she pushes herself and ignores the cold, which progresses to bronchitis and then pneumonia. She takes antibiotics, which don't help very much. Eventually, she recovers, but after that, she always feels fatigued. She just never seems to feel refreshed and rested. Now, Jane gets hot flashes and she sleeps poorly. She also begins to experience irregularities in her menstrual cycle. Sometimes she'll bleed for two weeks at a time, which, of course, is very alarming to her. She looks like she's beginning to exhibit the symptoms of perimenopause. Because of her symptoms and her age (she's now around forty-four), her Western doctor prescribes HRT. Not wanting to take this step, Jane returns to her TCM practitioner determined to find a way to get rid of her symptoms, and stay healthy without hormones. Because she has had a little bit of experience in self-healing over the past few decades, she knows she has to take this step seriously and take responsibility for her own health.

Jane now embarks on a journey of acupuncture, classical Chinese herbal therapy, and resumes her yoga and meditation classes. She makes different choices in the foods she eats and begins to eat for healing. She changes her workspace by adding plants and making it a more healthful environment. She lets go of a lot of anger and stress. Luckily, she can even talk with the people she works with to let them know that she is as productive as ever, but needs to draw some boundaries around her work schedule so that she does not expend too much energy. She and her husband and children work out a better distribution of chores. Jane now takes time and makes the effort to keep her emotions in balance. When she feels the least bit sick, she goes immediately to her TCM doctor and together they take care of the little things so that they don't escalate into full-blown conditions as her pneumonia did. Jane actually goes to her TCM doctor to stay well; twice a year she has an energy "tune-up" with acupuncture. Jane has begun to deeply appreciate the spiritual side of her that has emerged as she transforms her life and discovers her own self-healing ability. She's eager to share the wisdom that's come her way with many of her women friends. She finds deep peace and strength knowing that she is finally in charge of her own health.

CHAPTER 3

QI:
The Secret Behind
TCM

OFTEN when menopause patients first come to me, they tell me they've been to many different places to get well without good results. Usually, they come because their friend has urged them to make this appointment. They say: "I don't know why I'm here. I really hope you can help me because I've tried just about everything. What can TCM do for me?" I explain to them that what TCM can do is identify and treat the root cause of their problem, treat their body, mind, and spirit, and help them get their own healing ability to function strongly again. When we discuss treatment options, I tell them that I am not interested in covering up or suppressing their symptoms. I also tell them that TCM doesn't believe in cutting out problems unless absolutely necessary because unless the root cause is addressed, the problem still remains. We also talk about true prevention and its meaning. I tell them there is a big difference between doing healthy things on a daily basis to stay well and getting sick and going to the doctor to try and become well again.

I'll give you two examples of what I mean. If a woman has monthly menstrual cramps, what does she do? She takes one of the many over-the-counter painkillers every four to six hours for one or more days at a time. One of my patients told me she took at least twelve ibuprofen tablets during the first few days of her period for almost fifteen years.

Over time, the pills—as the package warned—gave her heartburn and stomach problems because her digestive system could no longer handle the painkilling drugs. She had not found a sustainable or healthy way to address her chronic symptoms. In fact, for fifteen years she had covered them up! Interestingly, she also compartmentalized these monthly occurrences. To her, they represented an ongoing inconvenience or, at certain times, chronic discomfort. By and large, however, this woman, who I might add was very intelligent, thought of herself overall as healthy, even though for one week out of the month—25 percent of each month—she was basically miserable!

Another example is a woman of menopausal age who is bleeding excessively. For a large majority of Western physicians, the treatment of choice would be to remove her uterus with a hysterectomy. While this may certainly clear up the excessive bleeding, it removes an organ that TCM sees as a "second engine" that generates Qi. Now, if one of the root causes of menopausal symptoms is a kidney Qi deficiency, then removing an important source of extra Qi does not appear to be preventive in nature. TCM thinks about these things differently.

TCM's healing practice is based on something even greater than the healing process itself—that is the Universe. TCM revolves around the concept that we are not isolated individuals, but rather, we are part of the greater Universal whole. We are, if you will, woven tightly into the web of the Universe. Therefore, it is within our grasp to get healing support from this greater force. To do so, a person's body has to be at its maximum function: that is, it has to be in harmony. Thus, the ultimate purpose of TCM is to find ways to keep the body in a condition of harmony and balance within itself so it can get more healing support from the larger Universe of which it's a part.

TCM's first line of thought, therefore, is not to mask symptoms like menstrual cramps and headaches that my patient had lived with for fifteen years, but rather to aggressively seek their source and deal with them at a deeper level so that the individual can return her system to a harmonious state. The same would be true for the menopausal woman who is bleeding heavily. A skillful doctor of TCM would first stop the bleeding, then immediately treat the root cause of the problem. Assuming, there is no cancer or tumors, TCM says the real cause of this condition is a function disorder of the spleen. It is too weak to perform its job of controlling the blood flow in the body. In this case, removing the uterus does not come close to addressing the root cause of the bleeding and would not be considered a healthy option.

For a long time, the prevailing thinking in the West has been that the uterus is no longer necessary for menopausal women. In the early 1990s, by the age of sixty, more than one-third of American women had had hysterectomies. After Cesarean sections, hysterectomies are the second most commonly performed operation. Among Western countries, the United States has the highest rate of hysterectomies; Norway, Sweden, and the United Kingdom have the lowest.

TCM sees things very differently. It believes that the uterus still has value, even though it does not produce the same amount of hormones that it did in the past. Why should it? There is no reason that a fifty-year-old woman (who no longer is bearing children) should need to generate the same amount of hormones as a twenty-eight-year-old. It goes against nature. And as we've noted, TCM views a person's body as woven into the web of nature and the Universe.

Here's a perspective on how TCM looks at this organ. Think about your grandmother and all the nice things she did with you when you were young. Your grandmother may have lived with your family all your life. She may have taken care of you and your brothers and sisters when you were children. She probably helped with the chores, and baby-sat when she was needed. Now, because she's older and perhaps not as strong as she used to be, she can do a lot less than when you were younger. But, you wouldn't kick her out of the house just because she could no longer do the same jobs she could previously. You still consider her a valued family member and she still maintains important relationships and communications with your other family members. Her loss would be felt by everyone. The same is true of any organ in your body. This is particularly true for a woman and her uterus. Nothing in your body lives an independent life; everything is connected through Qi.

TCM uses three main theories to correct a person's imbalance. These philosophical concepts have been in place for more than five thousand years. While there are other principles that can also be used to find the cause and solution for an individual's problem, these three are Universal truths that TCM practitioners use to guide their healing work. All Chinese art forms such as Taiji and other martial arts, bamboo painting, and Feng Shui (FUNG SHWAY), the art of place and placement, are all based on these theories. Although the world has radically changed since these principles were revealed, the Universal truths remain constant. They never change. These three major principles are: Qi and blood, yin and yang, and the Five Element Theory. I'm going to tell you, in turn, about each of them. It's important for me to provide this foundation of knowledge to help you understand the dynamics that create menopausal symptoms and what you can do about them. More importantly, these three principles will open up real knowledge that can help you tap into your own spirit so that it can come forward and flourish during this time of transformation.

UNDERSTANDING QI

While I frequently use the word Qi and energy interchangeably, there is a difference. I like to describe energy as a computer without any software. The hardware, of course, is visible and it's easy for us to see that it exists. You can touch it, but without software, it cannot function. It can't do anything useful for you without its internal programs. On the other hand, Qi is like a computer that comes with software. How many programs are loaded and up and running depends on you and how healthy you are.

The *Nei Jing* tells us that Qi is the root of all things. This ancient text also said that there are three related Qis: the Qi of heaven, the Qi of earth, and the Qi of humanity. The Qi of heaven represents the Universe and its "cosmic" energy. The Qi of earth is the "force of nature," and Qi of humanity is our own "life force." Without Qi and its animating force, there is nothing. For instance, when we die, our physical body remains, but our life force—our Qi—is gone. Whether you believe that this force exists or not, or has influence on your whole being or not, it does. You experience Qi every moment of your life. Qi is a real Universal force like wind, magnetics, gravity, and the speed of the earth's rotation. Though you may not be able to see it directly, you can see its effect everywhere in every moment. For example, the opening of a flower involves Qi; the ebb and flow of the ocean's tide is caused by Qi. Everything has Qi—animate and inanimate.

Classical Chinese medicine understands that there is a life force and it understands how to manipulate this force for healing purposes. Qi is also the means by which everything is connected and communicates with each other. Have you ever wondered why you feel so wonderful and so connected to the world around when you stand on a mountaintop overlooking the countryside? It is Qi that passes this "information" and "feeling" to you. Likewise, have you ever stood beside the magnificent California Redwood trees or large inanimate objects such as the giant stone pillars at Stonehenge in England? Or the Pyramids in Egypt? When you do, somewhere inside yourself, you realize that nature—even huge stones—has power. It makes sense. Those Redwoods and Stonehenge megaliths and the Pyramids have thousands of years of accumulated history and power, and it is Qi that communicates and connects their power to you. If you have ever been in their presence, you know just what I mean. We can connect with Qi either visually or through the invisible.

SEASONAL QI

TCM understands that everything has Qi—the sun, the moon, the earth, and all things, both living and nonliving. Even the seasons have their own Qi. Look at the differences between each of the seasons. I'm referring to the smells, sounds, sights, and general feeling of the various times of the year. Nature itself certainly understands these differences. You probably have recognized the uniqueness of seasonal energies too if you've ever tried planting something out of its normal season. Whatever you put in the ground may grow (especially if you live in a climate with mild winters), but it may never flower or bear fruit. That's because the planting process for this particular thing was out of sync with its proper seasonal Qi.

Whether we perceive it or not, each season's Qi exerts an influence on our bodies and in our lives. So it's important for us to be synchronous with a season's flow. Unfortunately, given our busy lives where we run from morning until night, we barely notice the changing leaves let alone the changing Qi. As a result, many people get sick when the seasons change. Most attribute their illnesses to changes in the temperature, or "catching" something from someone else. The real cause is quite different.

TCM says that one of the reasons that disease or illness occurs is because a person's Qi cannot match or adjust smoothly to the Qi of the new season. Many people experience health problems, such as hay fever in the spring or the fall, when seasonal changes occur. If they cannot weather these seasonal changes successfully, these problems can linger and go much deeper. For example, we often see a lot of people catch a cold and develop a cough during the fall, which is the season of the lung. If this cough doesn't get fixed completely during the fall, it can evolve into more serious conditions like bronchitis or pneumonia during winter.

If you find that you get sick when seasonal changes occur, you should understand that your body's Qi is either out of balance, or what TCM calls deficient. Your overall Qi either is too low, or a specific organ's Qi does not have enough power to perform the job that it was created to do. Another factor could be that your organs are not working in harmony. Healthy people do not get hay fever or allergies. It is more useful to look internally for the answer to your health problems rather than externally and think that the pollen from your neighbor's trees and flowers, or the hair or dander of dogs and cats, has caused your discomforts. If you already have a serious health problem, you should take especially good care of yourself during seasonal changes. If you are in perimenopause and experiencing intermittent symptoms such as PMS, migraine headaches, digestive problems, etc., you should be especially careful around the time of seasonal changes. Likewise, women who have menopausal symptoms must take extra good care of themselves around these times.

In the Five Element Theory (which is explained in greater detail in Chapter 5), TCM teaches us that each of our five organs is related to one of the seasons. TCM recognizes a fifth season called Late Summer, which relates to the spleen. Each organ is particularly prone to problems during its season. However, if we are aware of how things really work, we can cooperate with the seasonal changes and use them to strengthen our overall health and that of each season's related organ. We can do this by eating the right foods and herbs, wearing the proper clothes, and doing Qigong movements to increase Qi. Unfortunately, most people of the West don't know this and often, as the seasons change, experience problems in the organs that are related to that specific time of year. Spring, for example, is the season of the liver. It is a time when nature's Qi is rising, causing seeds to germinate and plants to grow. In your body, liver Qi rises in the spring as well. However, if your liver Qi rises too forcefully in the spring, it can cause problems, like hypertension, migraine headaches, mood swings, and more. The purpose of riding each season's energy changes is preventive in nature. Imagine how much less stress and wear and tear you put on your body when you avoid a constant progression of illnesses and diseases. You are beginning to understand how to save your precious healing Qi to live a long, healthy life—TCM's most important goal.

Here's an example of what I mean. One of my patients, Susan, came to see me in May several years ago because she had a continuous headache that throbbed at the top of her head that began in late March. I knew immediately that her problem was caused by a liver dysfunction because spring can bring on headaches, especially on the top of the head where the liver meridian runs. This season's Qi can also cause anger, bad moods, and mood swings if liver Qi cannot flow smoothly. Together we worked to rebalance her liver function with herbs, Qigong movements, and lifestyle changes that she was very committed to making.

Summer is the season of heat and relates to the heart. The Qi of summer is hot, and very big and inflated. Many heart problems occur as a result of an excess of heat in this organ. That is why I always tell my patients to avoid broiling in the sun. The excess heat can cause enormous damage both on the surface of the skin and internally.

As we've said, the lung is related to autumn Qi. If your own Qi cannot ride this season's energy change or make a smooth transition with its Qi, you will be very vulnerable to coughs and colds. Perhaps you've noticed that you and your children in particular get stubborn coughs beginning in late September. That's because the seasonal Qi is diminishing and beginning to pull in. It is a dry energy. As a result, the lung, which is the source for these coughs and colds, gets dry as well. If you can keep your Qi and that of your children's balanced and strong and keep your organs working in harmony, you will not be affected by external pathogens, no matter what time of year.

Winter is the season of the kidney. The Qi of winter is closed and quiet, and small and slow. This Qi needs to be protected and stored up for the following spring. It is a time of year when people should also take it more slowly and not schedule too many activities. But once again, given our busy Western lifestyles, most of us don't stop the whirlwind we live in. Think about the procession of holidays and holy days from Halloween through midnight before the New Year! Who is slowing down in this season? Virtually no one. As a result, during the cold months of the year, kidney Qi, the foundation of your very life force, gets depleted rather than quietly stored. Infections of all kinds tend to occur in this season as well.

In January, it's no wonder I see so many Western patients who are sick. After shopping and partying from late November through December, and on into the New Year, they have used up enormous reserves of Qi to keep going. They don't realize it, but this level of activity is in direct opposition to the natural Qi or energetic force of winter. No wonder they're exhausted! The Qi they needed for "a long winter's nap," is gone. If they're relatively healthy, they might feel merely tired or fatigued after the holidays. But, if they're not so healthy, they may experience an illness or old symptoms may recur every year. For example, I find that some of my menopause patients are able to eliminate virtually all of their discomforts or symptoms before the holidays. After the holidays, all our good work is undone, because their hot flashes, night sweats, and mood swings, among other symptoms, return. Why? Because they have depleted their organs' Qi and these organs cannot perform the functions ingrained in them, nor can they work in harmony with each other. If you add a problem of Qi stagnation anywhere in the body, you will definitely have a recurrence of menopausal symptoms.

Now that you are aware of the direct relationship between menopausal symptoms and weak kidney Qi, you shouldn't be surprised when I tell you that winter can especially be hard on women who are ages forty and up. They often feel tired and low. If women and older people (who also suffer from weak Qi) are sick during the winter, I almost always find that the root cause is impaired kidney function. While summer and winter seasonal changes can affect people with heart disease, winter has a much more serious affect. People with these conditions should pay particular attention to conserving Qi during the winter. We will discuss this in more detail in the Five Element Theory.

In evaluating my patients' conditions, it is essential that I factor in the time of year when diagnosing their health issues. A well-trained TCM doctor always considers the effect of the current seasonal change, no matter whether the patient's condition is acute or chronic.

QI IN THE ORGANS

TCM sees the human body as a microcosm of the Universe. Thus, the Qi of humanity resides within us as Inborn Qi and Acquired Qi. Yet if we looked under a microscope and tried to "see" Qi, we would not find it. But it's there. Quantum physicists know it's there, because they have a deeper insight into these kinds of forces that integrate well with quantum theories.

As I've noted, each of the body's organs has its own Qi. TCM says that the organs and all functions of our body and mind communicate with each other via Qi and the meridians. The example I often like to use is that internally, you are a very busy switchboard abuzz with constant messages about the state of your health! These messages are virtually uncountable and zip through your body at immeasurable speeds.

Imagine, if you will, the inner workings of your body. Inside

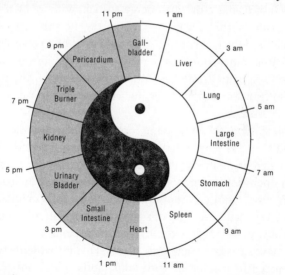

TWENTY-FOUR HOUR QI OR ENERGY CLOCK

(Each organ is in charge of the body during its two-hour watch.)

are meridians or energy pathways that connect every part of the body, as well as its interior with the exterior. They enable the body to work as a coherent unit. It is because of meridians that acupuncture and acupressure have their effect. As we'll see in Chapter 10, the flow of Qi through your meridians can be enhanced or modified either with acupuncture needles or with the hands through acupressure massage. This means that problems inside your body can be fixed from the outside.

Recently, the National Institutes of Health (NIH) acknowledged the mechanism of meridians and the flow of Qi in its "Consensus Development Conference Statement on Acupuncture" and its acceptance of the efficacy of acupuncture for certain health conditions: "The general theory of acupuncture is based on the premise that there are patterns of energy flow (Qi) through the body that are essential for health. Disruptions of this flow are believed to be responsible for disease."

Each of us has a unique energy system, with its own operating program. Within the system, there are the subsystems of organs, each of which is controlled by an aspect of a person's spirit. The spiritual dimension of a person is vitally important in TCM. A person's spiritual state has enormous bearing on the person's ability to transform themselves, to self-heal, and to recover from illness or disease.

The spirit is the organizing force that tells an organ how to function. That is why organ transplants are often rejected. The transplanted organ brings its own spirit and its own message from another operating energy system. When you hook it up to another person's power and program, there is a fairly good chance that it could be rejected. Each organ's messages are different and they cannot always be integrated into the new system.

When discussing organ transplants, I tell my patients they can be compared to moving in with your mother- and father-in-law. Sure, you may get along with your husband (or partner) all right, but now you need to build a relationship with your in-laws. Living in such close quarters can be very challenging! Some people can get along; others fight like cats and dogs and find this situation unbearable, and eventually reject the relationship altogether. It is the same with an organ transplant. If you're lucky, it works.

Again, let me emphasize these concepts. It is through Qi and meridians that our life-giving organs communicate with one another. So whenever there is an energy problem with one of the organs, our entire system is affected. Like a television, the body needs power—it has to be plugged in, but all the parts on the inside also have to function well. The organs are like the different channels, each with its own frequency. If the frequency of any of the channels is off, or weak, or can't be received, the television won't work well. It's the same with our bodies. TCM recognizes that problems in one area will affect the workings of the whole; in this medical system, treating parts in isolation is not the answer.

If an organ's Qi is excessive or deficient, an organ dysfunction will result. Then another organ will be affected, then another, and so forth. Since they're all connected through Qi all the time, it's a serious matter to have an organ fall out of balance. It then opens the way for a domino effect, where one organ after another can be affected to one degree or another. I think a lot of people reading this book may have been through this kind of loop. But this situation might make even more sense when you view it from the TCM perspective. Consequently, it's very important for a good TCM practitioner to go beyond the symptoms and identify the true source of any health problem, especially minor ones before they can cause bigger problems. In TCM, prevention truly is the cure.

For example, my patient, Lily, came to me to help her with stomach problems. Her symptoms were a tongue with a greasy, yellow coating, bad breath, stomach distention, and constipation. Her nose was also very red, she had bleeding gums, and a condition called temporomandibular joint dysfunction (TMJ), which caused her great pain when she moved her jaw to eat or speak.

Although it might seem that the root cause of Lily's problem was her stomach, that was not the case: it was her liver. Lily is an investment banker, a wife, and mother of two young boys. She was constantly traveling and juggling her busy schedule. She told me that she often felt frustrated that she never seemed to have time for anything.

I explained to her that being in a chronic state of anger and continually being under such tremendous stress had caused her to develop a liver function disorder. In this case, the flow of her liver Qi had been disrupted and become stuck in her stomach. With this condition, the liver generates excessive heat, which is then passed on to the stomach, where it stagnates. This, in turn, caused her stomach pain, distention, acid indigestion, etc. She explained she had indeed tried everything possible to alleviate her stomach discomfort, but nothing seemed to work. I told her that the real problem was a liver function disorder and that unless this was treated, her stomach problems could not heal. I gave her herbs, taught her several Qigong movements or meridian stretches, and stressed how important it was for her to slow down and change her lifestyle.

Although her stomach problems improved greatly, Lily's schedule, if anything, has become even busier. Therefore, she must continue being treated and cannot hope to see 100 percent improvement—unless she decides to live life at a slower, less demanding pace.

I watch so many Western women struggle with the concept of slowing down. They have so many demands on them, often they cannot see a way to relinquish their endless chores and obligations. Actually, we spend a lot of time discussing this. Repeatedly, I ask them how can they put their own life and health in second place? How will their families fare if they are in poor health or struggling daily with chronic health problems? These are questions I hope you will ask yourself before you are affected by menopausal symptoms. Lily is not unusual; over many years of practice, I have seen so many Western women like her complain of stomach problems, often accompanied by headaches, including migraines, especially after eating. Although the seriousness of their problems vary greatly, I always tell them that to truly heal these conditions, they must change their lifestyles. The effectiveness of my treatment really depends on their willingness to cooperate.

If, as in Lily's case, liver Qi gets out of control, it goes to places it shouldn't, such as to the stomach. TCM theory states that uncontrolled liver Qi causes too much internal movement. Western doctors might see these symptoms of involuntary movements on the surface and call it a motor issue. An example would be Parkinson's disease where a person is constantly shaking or in motion. A TCM practitioner would diagnose the root cause of this condition as a liver function disorder, rather than a problem of the brain. TCM treatment would focus on bringing liver function back into balance and restoring harmony with the other organs.

As a TCM practitioner, it is my responsibility to do what I can to help each of my patients discover and revitalize her Qi, and to ensure that it flows smoothly. Here's another key principle relating to the all-important Qi.

QI AND BLOOD: INTERTWINED RIVERS OF LIFE

While the concept of Qi and blood is complex, it is a crucial one. Some people may have experience with this concept. It helps explain why and how a TCM practitioner can diagnose and treat disease and illness. This concept also helps clarify why TCM believes that forcing the menstrual cycle to continue after it should stop is not only unnatural, but unhealthy.

In TCM theory, blood is the "mother" of Qi. Like any good mother, it carries Qi and gives it its material form. It also provides nutrients for its movement. The *Nei Jing* tells us:

> *Blood is the mother of Qi.*
> *Qi is the commander of the blood.*

So while blood is the "mother" of Qi, Qi is the "commander" of the blood. This means that Qi is the force that both makes blood flow throughout the body and guides it to the places it needs to be. Blood and Qi are inextricably entwined and each affects the other. They cannot be separated. To put it another way, without the blood, the formless Qi has no place to reside. On the other hand, without the power and intelligence of Qi, the blood has no life force, nor can it determine where it must flow. One cannot survive without the other. They also have control over one another. Within this closest of relationships, blood and Qi have the dynamic ability to transfer various properties back and forth.

Therefore, if your Qi is deficient, you will also have deficient blood and vice versa. For instance, spotting between menstrual cycles, if there is no tumor or internal bleeding, is regarded by TCM as a serious sign that your Qi is deficient. In this case, because Qi is deficient, it cannot do its job of making sure blood flows normally. In fact without proper Qi, blood flow—which is why uncontrolled bleeding from the uterus, the gums, nose, even hemophilia— is directly related to the relationship between Qi and blood. If blood is deficient, the body's internal environment cannot be balanced nor well-nourished. That's why spotting causes fatigue or insomnia and weight loss.

After childbirth, for example, women sometimes experience a low-grade fever. From the TCM point of view, this is caused by blood deficiency, not by an infection. TCM would counteract this condition by increasing a woman's Qi or increasing her blood through special herbs and foods. For this condition, ginseng is one of the best herbs to increase Qi and help reduce fever. TCM would not prescribe antibiotics, because it does believe the source of the fever is an infection. Deficient blood can also play a role in other problems, such as various menstrual disorders, heart palpitations, and insomnia, to name a few.

For menopausal women, it's important to know that TCM states that the liver is the storehouse of blood. This organ also governs the flow of Qi throughout the body, smoothing and regulating the circulation of both blood and its inseparable companion Qi.

The *Nei Jing* describes the liver as "the root of stopping all extremes." Let me explain what this means.

If the flow of Qi or blood becomes blocked or stagnates, it is the liver's function to free it up again. However, as I explained in the Introduction, when women reach menopausal age, their liver function is usually sluggish or poor. This condition, you know by now, is often the result of stress and the physical and emotional challenges of everyday life. So if a woman's liver function is poor, Qi and blood can stagnate. For menopausal women, this problem can cause insomnia, spotting, blood in the urine, urinary tract infections, as well as frequent urination.

Because the main function of the liver is that of free flow, it is also the organ most sensitive to problems of stagnation (of Qi, blood, and even emotions). The liver is also prone to problems of excess when its energy becomes hyperactive and flares up. This happens most easily in the liver's season, the spring, when nature's own Qi, as we've discussed, is rising up as well. When the liver's energy rises up too forcefully, you may suffer from headaches, dizziness, irritability, or hypertension. If the liver is functioning as it should, however, it will "stop" these extremes by relaxing the excessive flow of Qi that is moving too strongly through the body. That is the meaning of the *Nei Jing*'s statement about the role the liver plays as the "root of stopping all extremes."

The liver also has an important relationship with the spleen, which is the organ that transforms food from the stomach into Qi and blood. It plays a vital role in maintaining good digestion. If the spleen does not get the necessary support from the liver because this organ is not functioning well, the spleen will not be able to transform food into Qi and blood. If the transformation process doesn't occur smoothly, health problems will surface. For example, an individual with spleen and liver problems tends to bruise easily. This occurs because the liver is not doing its job of circulating the blood. The blood, in turn, begins to pool or stagnate under the skin. In this situation, the relationship between the spleen and the liver is functioning poorly. So every time the person's skin is touched or hit, a bruise (which is coagulated blood) can appear. Also, an individual with deficient liver Qi and blood can have dry, cracked, and brittle nails—a common problem among older people who are prone to problems of liver function.

And as you'll see further in The Five Element Theory, TCM

considers the eyes as the "opening" of the liver. Therefore, people with deficient liver blood can also experience problems with their eyes such as dryness, burning, and blurred or deteriorating vision. Because the eyes are the doorway to the liver, the reverse is also true: too much "looking" hurts the liver. Computers are a fact of life for so many women, but if you spend a great deal of time at the computer, you should understand the health consequences. Those long, uninterrupted hours in front of the computer are not good for you. Not just because they make you tired. The health of your liver is at stake. This kind of overuse of the eyes can actually drain your liver Qi—another unforeseen problem of modern life. To help yourself, I recommend having green plants in your workspace. Resting and relieving your eyes by looking at something fresh, green, and alive several times throughout the day, can actually make a big difference over time.

Some menopausal women suffer from joint pain, and this, too, relates to liver Qi, which governs the tendons and ligaments. Many joint problems are often related to tendon problems. The joints depend on sufficient blood from the liver to nourish the tendons and ligaments so that they function properly. A lot of women don't realize it but they have harmed their tendons and liver by overexercising. Overexercising is a bigger problem for women than for men because the liver is the most important organ for women's health. (For men, the most important is the kidney.) Excessive aerobics and jogging, for example, are both very bad for the tendons, which are like rubber bands. If you overstretch them, they become too loose and flexibility is lost. Women who do a lot of aerobics or who run too much, can actually drain their liver Qi. If they really overdo it, they may stop getting their periods, get tendonitis, or end up (in extreme cases) with chronic fatigue syndrome.

QI DEFICIENCY

The condition of Qi deficiency can be debilitating. Your body can suffer from an overall deficiency of Qi, or you can have a Qi deficiency of a specific organ. In either case, it means your body or a particular organ (or organs) has insufficient power to do its proper job. When Qi is deficient, your entire body stops functioning well. Problems stemming from deficient overall Qi can cause a lot of physical discomfort and distress—like constant headaches, bad moods, poor digestion, nausea, insomnia, to name a few. If this happens, your medical and scientific tests might still be normal. Yet don't be fooled. This is the very time you should become alert to the fact that your organs are sending you an SOS. They're telling you, "Help! We are falling out of balance! We really need some attention!" This is definitely the time to take preventive actions to safeguard your precious energy system; this is not a time to ignore the internal messages your body is sending.

Quite often women with deficient Qi are told by their physicians that there is no physical basis for their complaints and discomfort. TCM practitioners would disagree. We see many of these complaints and discomforts and recognize them as a deficiency in Qi. Oftentimes, these conditions point to kidney Qi deficiency—a very serious matter. Remember, this is because your Inborn Qi stored in the kidney is limited and cannot be replenished. And as I said earlier, when Inborn Qi has been used up, it's time to leave this earth.

In my practice, many Western women walk into my office very apologetic about their condition because they have no real medical proof. They say, "I don't think I'm *that* sick, but I really don't feel well. Maybe I just need a rest?" They're always surprised when I tell them: "I don't need to see your blood tests or your x-rays, or your CT scans, or your MRI results. I need to look at you and do a pulse diagnosis. Most important, I need to talk with you. I need to pay attention to who you really are." I tell them not to worry about having something wrong with them, that their problem may be beyond physical science, but it is definitely not without cause. I also reassure these really wonderful women that they are not crazy and do not need to see a psychiatrist. I am amazed at how many of them tell me that they have basically been dismissed by modern medicine because their test results are normal. Often, they start crying because, at last, they have encoun-

tered a medical system that understands their discomfort and
pain and can diagnose and help relieve these conditions.

DAILY CYCLE OF QI

Certain problems may also appear, or worsen, at specific times of
day. This has to do with the daily cycle of Qi among the twelve organs. TCM theory explains that Universal energy changes every
two hours and your body's meridian and organ energies respond
to and match these changes. In other words, each organ has a two-
hour period when it is "on duty" or in charge of your body. During this particular time, the organ on duty is like a traffic director
overseeing the flow and activities of the entire body. If that organ,
or director, is out to lunch or not functioning well, havoc can
break loose with traffic jams as bothersome and serious as those
on a thruway during rush hour!

TCM practitioners have worked with this theory for many
centuries and know when each organ is on duty. They use this information to diagnose a possible problem with that organ. For example, the chart below shows that the lung is in charge of the
body from 3:00 to 5:00 A.M. If you find yourself waking up between these hours with any physical discomfort including nightmares, it could be a sign that your lung Qi is weak or deficient.
Likewise, if you are bothered by any problem at 5:00 P.M., for example diarrhea, it could be a problem with your kidney Qi. In this
instance, I might treat your spleen (to deal with the diarrhea)
with herbs, but I would also add another herb (or herbs) to
strengthen your kidney Qi as well.

DAILY CYCLE WHEN QI PEAKS

Lung   3:00 A.M.–5:00 A.M.
Large intestine 5:00 A.M.–7:00 A.M.
Spleen   7:00 A.M.–9:00 A.M.
Stomach   9:00 A.M.–11:00 A.M.

Heart	11:00 A.M.–1:00 P.M.
Small intestine	1:00 P.M.–3:00 P.M.
Bladder	3:00 P.M.–5:00 P.M.
Kidney	5:00 P.M.–7:00 P.M.
Pericardium	7:00 P.M.–9:00 P.M.
Triple warmer	9:00 P.M.–11:00 P.M.
Gallbladder	11:00 P.M.–1:00 A.M.
Liver	1:00 A.M.–3:00 A.M.

Time is a very important clue for the TCM doctor. So as you can see, Qi is one important way doctors of TCM diagnose and treat illnesses. Remember, we see disease as an energy or function problem. Western medicine at the present time has not figured how to evaluate TCM's five-thousand-year-old practice using its existing scientific measurements. However, quantum physicists who also work with energy and must base their information on more than observation alone, are very much in tune with our ancient knowledge. They know there is Qi out there and within us, and that these two energies are linked—what we call the Universal Qi and the Qi of humanity.

Everything responds to Qi. Here's an interesting story of how animals respond to it. For example, several years ago, four thousand homing pigeons were released in New Jersey during a regular race. Do you know that not one of them found their way back home? Do you know why? It is not familiar landmarks that direct these amazing birds, but rather it is the unseen magnetic energy, or Qi, of the earth that allows them to find their way back home. And when these energies experience shifts or disturbances, as they did at that time because of the effects of a major solar storm, the pigeons' tracking systems no longer function properly. In these cases, they literally lose their connection with the Qi of the earth and become confused. Everything is about Qi or energy.

You know, many people these days spend a lot of money at a health spa to improve their body, mind, and spirit. How do you think these three elements connect to each other within one human being? In TCM, we believe the connection is through Qi. And a good TCM practitioner can use his or her Qi to interact with yours and provide you with the proper treatments to help you heal yourself and help you integrate your own body, mind, and spirit. That is what I hope you will learn from the ancient wisdom in this book.

In the next chapter, I am going to tell you about the magic and the miracle that is called yin and yang.

TO SUMMARIZE:

- Qi is the life force that animates all things. It is everywhere and in everything.
- Qi and blood have a profound and inseparable relationship: blood is the mother of Qi and Qi is its commander.
- A good TCM doctor always applies the concept of Qi to diagnose and treat a person's problem or condition.
- Seasonal Qi influences our bodies and health.
- Each of our five major organs has its own Qi and each organ is related to a specific season. If an organ cannot make a smooth energy transition with a new season, health problems often arise at that time.
- In evaluating patients' conditions, a good TCM doctor always takes into account the time of year it is.
- Each organ has a two-hour period during the day when its Qi is the strongest. Experiencing problems during specific times of the day indicates a problem with its corresponding organ.
- Western medicine has no way to measure Qi and no way to understand its relationship to healthy organ function.
- In menopausal women, poor liver function (often caused by chronic anger, stress, and certain lifestyle habits) can cause problems with the blood and Qi such as joint pain and tendon problems.

Yang Qi looks like heaven and the sun.
Without it, life is depleted and vibrant growth comes
with struggle.

Yang Qi movement is like the brilliance of the sun
Therefore, yang Qi radiates above and outside of all
things.

NEI JING (475–221 B.C.)

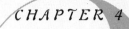

CHAPTER 4

The Complementary Dance of Yin and Yang Energies

*T*CM believes everything is composed of two complementary energies; one energy is yin (EEN) and the other is yang (YAHN). They are never separate; one cannot exist without the other. TCM defines this as the Yin/Yang Theory of Opposition and Interdependence. This intertwined and inseparable relationship is reflected in the circular yin/yang symbol seen above. Look carefully at this symbol; no matter where you divide this circle in half, the divided section always contains the Qi, or energy, of both yin and yang—even if it is just one small dot. Just like Qi and blood, they are indivisible and inseparable.

The ancient Chinese masters did not make up the Theory of Yin/Yang; they were able to identify and observe the interplay of these energies in a way that we really can't today. Yin and yang are a part of the natural law. Age-old TCM texts say that "if you understand yin and yang, you can hold the Universe in your hands." These two Universal energies are in everything, including our bodies. Everything can be divided into yin and yang. Here are some examples:

YIN	YANG
Female	Male
Water	Fire
Cold	Hot
Interior	Exterior
Slow	Fast
Contraction	Expansion
Passive	Active
Deficiency	Excess
Moon	Sun
Night	Day

Because these energies are dynamic, or always moving, the Theory of Yin/Yang contains no absolutes. The designation of something as yin or yang is always relative to, or in comparison with, some other thing. For example, the sun and daytime are considered to be yang in relation to the moon and the night. But within daytime, early morning is yin compared with noon; and within the night, the full moon is yang compared with the darkness of the sky, and so on. As we've seen, even within yang, yin energy is present; within yin, there is still yang energy. They not only oppose each other, but are interdependent as well. You cannot have one without the other. That's the beauty of yin and yang. This is Universal law at its simplest and deepest. According to this theory, yang is male; yin is female. But that is not to say that men just have yang problems and female just have yin conditions. It is a generalization that gives you an overall sense of the differences between the two energies.

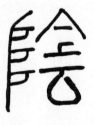

Yin

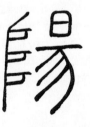

Yang

Everything in the body is also under the control of yin and yang. For example, the front of your body is yin; the back of your body is yang. Your head is yang; your feet are yin. The outside of your arms and legs are yang, but the inside is considered yin. Internally, Qi is yang; blood and body fluids are yin. The five major organs or viscera (liver, heart, spleen, lung, kidney) are yin; their respective partner organs (gallbladder, small intestine, stomach, large intestine, and bladder—called bowels in TCM), are yang.

Because yin and yang have an inseparable relationship, you can see that if you have a problem with one, the other will also have a problem. If your gallbladder suffers from an imbalance, sooner or later, it will affect the liver, its corresponding partner, or vice versa. It's also important to understand that despite their specific yin/yang designation, each of the organs listed above also have yin and yang energies within themselves, and these energies must also remain in harmony. When you consider these fundamental energies and the job of keeping them not only balanced, but in harmony as well, you can begin to appreciate the amazingly complex, yet delicate task of keeping these dynamic systems in equilibrium for your body, mind, and spirit to remain well.

Why does TCM consider this theory so important to good health? Western medicine tends to look at your numbers: your blood pressure, your high-density lipoprotein (HDL), and low-density lipoprotein (LDL) cholesterol numbers, your heart rate, pulse rate, among others. If your numbers are good, you are pronounced healthy. You may not feel healthy (in fact, you might feel very much the opposite), but the numbers appear to indicate you are healthy. Within the context of Western medicine, it is difficult to take your problems any further if your numbers are normal.

TCM has a different perspective. It sees you as an infinite number of relationships that must remain not just in balance, but in harmony. When a TCM practitioner perceives that you are in this state, he or she knows you are healthy. More to the point, *you* know you are healthy. No one has to tell you that you are.

Let's look at a car analogy: You can own a brand new car, but if you've bought a "lemon," it just won't function properly. Your neighbor can own a ten-year-old car and, because he's maintained it lovingly over the past decade, it still runs quite well. Maybe it's not as fast as it used to be, but it's reliable, it's solid, and it never breaks down.

It's the same way with individuals as they age. Older people can live healthy lives when the relationships of their organs are balanced and their yin and yang energies are in harmony. Even though they cannot perform strenuous physical activities, they eat well, they sleep well, their emotions are balanced, they are happy always and they don't need to take an endless array of medications. For their age, they are in a state of excellent health. Contrast this with people who are much younger. Even though they have youth on their side, they can actually be less healthy than the older people we just talked about. They may suffer from indigestion problems, run themselves ragged every day, work sixty hours or more a week, and suffer from depression. They also may take large quantities of over-the-counter medications, or even drugs. Who is healthy and who is balanced? When you begin to grasp these concepts, you can see how your body really works and why certain things that we do in the West that we believe keep us healthy, are really detrimental to our well being.

YIN	YANG
Front of body	Back of body
Feet	Head
Inside of arms and legs	Outside of arms and legs
Blood and fluids	Qi
Liver	Gallbladder
Heart	Small intestine
Spleen	Stomach
Lung	Large intestine
Kidney	Bladder

TCM has an ancient saying: "As long as you know the theory of yin and yang, you can be a good TCM doctor." The energies of yin and yang are the basis of the most fundamental method of

TCM diagnosis. For thousands of years, TCM practitioners have regarded all disease or imbalances in terms of eight possible problems, which it calls the Eight Principal Syndromes. According to this TCM theory, yin/yang is the key to this.

EIGHT PRINCIPAL SYNDROMES

Yin	Yang
Cold	Heat
Interior	Exterior
Deficiency	Excess

In TCM, proper diagnosis of the root cause is everything. For instance, if I start by diagnosing a condition from the point of view of yin and yang, I can already achieve a 50 percent chance of being correct. Its root cause is either a yin energy problem or it might be yang. Now, I can continue to improve the degree of correctness of my diagnosis and therefore treatment. Here I move on to take into consideration the other six principal syndromes (that is, if a problem is interior or exterior, created by cold or heat, suffers from a deficiency or excess). I also refine my insight further by using Qi and the Five Element Theory (which we'll discuss in greater depth in Chapter 5) to identify the cause of and treatment for a person's illness. Also, my training as a Qigong master allows me to bring my intuition to bear on each patient's problem.

According to the modern medical textbook used in today's TCM colleges, menopausal symptoms are almost always caused by a kidney yin or kidney yang Qi deficiency. Sometimes a woman can suffer from both. The textbook says that it may also be compounded by a function disorder of any one of these organs— heart, spleen, and liver. Through my many years of experience of treating Western women and from the special knowledge I received from my master, I believe it is essential to look at Western menopause differently. I discovered a simple, direct way to treat the root cause of this condition without going through the more

complex classical approach. I regard Western menopausal symptoms as a kidney Qi deficiency and a liver function disorder. I
have discovered that to treat these conditions effectively it is not
necessary to divide them further along the classical theories for
treatment to be successful.

Sometimes my patients ask me, "How do you know whether
to use yin/yang, Qi, or the Five Element Theory? How do you
know which techniques to use and when?" I always tell them that
understanding the TCM theories and techniques is essential, but
deeply skilled TCM practitioners have the ability to look beyond
these things and use their intuition. Here's one way to understand this. Basically, good chefs can cook anything. It's not just
the ingredients they put in; it's also *how* they cook. There's a certain inspiration and direction that they know is right for a certain
dish and they follow their intuition to create it. Like a good chef,
a good TCM practitioner doesn't need to remain at the theory or
technique level, he or she can soar beyond the fundamentals and
create their own new recipes. This is the practice of the *art* of
medicine.

A word about balance and harmony. Ideally, yin and yang
should always remain in harmony, not, as many people think, in
balance. The words balance and harmony are sometimes used interchangeably, but I would like you to understand that they are
quite different. Balance is merely the first step toward harmony.
Two things can be balanced; they can have equal weight in a scale
and yet still be separate. Harmony means that they are not just
equal, but blended into a seamless whole. This condition of harmony reflects a dynamic state where these energies wax and wane
automatically. When one predominates, the other recedes.

For instance, when too many days of summer heat build up,
nature will cool the earth down with thunderstorms. If Indian
summer occurs and the weather is too hot, eventually nature will
create rainy weather; inevitably cooler days will follow. These
same dynamics of yin and yang energies continually occur within
your body. When this happens smoothly, you are healthy. If for
any reason, the energies become unbalanced, your health suffers.

Let's go a little more deeply into this concept. Balance has to do with the relationship between two separate entities: the relationship between you and me, for instance, or the relationship between your heart and your kidney. In your body, each organ itself must function or do its job properly, then its relationship with other organs must be balanced. Once they're in balance, the next step is to achieve harmony. As we've seen with the yin/yang symbol, when two things are in harmony, their energies blend together. Exchanges between things that are in balance have to be "manual," like going to the bank to transfer money from one account to another. However, if I've made certain arrangements in advance and the system is operating correctly, then I don't have to physically get in my car and go to my bank to transfer money, it will happen automatically.

When two things are in harmony, there is an ongoing, unconscious dance between them that happens naturally. In other words, in a healthy system, an "automatic transfer" happens—both within the body itself and between the body and the outside forces of nature to which it's connected. For example, as we've seen, when nature's Qi changes, your internal Qi responds automatically. When the seasons change like summer into fall, your internal Qi should automatically readjust itself to match nature's new energy frequency. If you can't make this switch smoothly, that's when you get sick. This is not an intellectual concept. This is the way things work according to natural law. Working with natural law instead of working against it can make a world of difference in the state of your health. This is especially significant for women going through the transition of menopause.

The reason that it's important to know whether a problem arises from yin or yang conditions is that it always affects the choice of herbs or selection of treatment options. Let's now apply the yin/yang theory to the diagnosis and treatment of menopause.

One of my patients, Louisa, age fifty-three, was experiencing hot flashes. Almost always, I believe, hot flashes for Western women are problems of kidney Qi deficiency. This means that the whole body's Qi or energy level is too weak to carry on its normal activities. But, I needed to know more. The Theory of Yin/Yang provided my next step for looking deeper into her problem. So I asked Louisa a question that I often ask my patients: What time of day was she experiencing her symptoms? Specifically, I wanted to know if her hot flashes occurred more often during the night or daytime. She told me that they almost always happened during the day. During the daytime, yang energy is dominant. Therefore, her hot flashes belonged in the category of a "yang Qi deficiency." To treat her specific condition, I chose a combination of herbs with the ability to help boost the yang Qi of her kidney. Had her hot flashes occurred predominantly at night, they would most likely have been related to a yin Qi deficiency. In that case, I would have treated her condition differently and with different herbs.

Another patient, Barbara, age forty, was having extremely difficult menstrual cramps. She said that hot baths and a heating pad on her abdomen usually helped relieve some of the pain. According to the Theory of Yin/Yang, yang energy is related to warmth and heat. Because Barbara's condition improved with the application of heat, it meant that her internal environment had become unbalanced and was suffering from too much cold. She was therefore deficient in, or had too little yang Qi. The first thing we did was increase and strengthen her yang Qi to bring warmth to the interior of her body. In addition to herbs for her liver, I recommended that she add certain foods to her diet that have the capability of increasing internal warmth. I told her to drink warm soups and to also mix in foods like cinnamon, ginger, fennel, and clove, that carry a warm essence. I explained that these same ingredients could also be put together in a small pillow and placed over her womb because all these spices carry a warm essence and can bring physical and energy warmth and relief from painful or uncomfortable cramps. All of these treatments helped her greatly. They alleviated the presenting problem, but went beyond it to help rebalance the root cause. You can do the same thing for yourself. Be sure and see the recipes in Chapter 15.

Age is also related to yin and yang energies. Because everything is under this natural law, so are we. Each of our lives and our physical bodies are influenced by yin and yang. The BaGua diagram on page 24 is based on one of the key energy theories of the *I Ching* called Twelve Energies Transition Theory. Look at the diagram and think of it in terms of a woman's lifetime. The circle is divided into twelve equal sections. Each section represents a seven-year cycle in a woman's life. The very top represents the time before she first menstruates. At this moment, she is at the pinnacle of her yang Qi. Then slowly, as we go clockwise down the right side of the circle, yang Qi diminishes and yin Qi increases. This yang Qi depletion and yin Qi increase continues until the point at the bottom—which is the 6th cycle, a woman's 42nd year, when she is almost at menopausal age. At this time, she becomes all yin Qi. You can see that she is missing any yang Qi influence or help. This is not a healthy balanced state in which she can remain for long without some sort of assistance.

TCM believes that it is vital to build up a woman's yang Qi before she reaches this point. If she can do this, if she can go through this transitional window, then she has the opportunity to revitalize herself. If this yang Qi buildup can take place, she will never need HRT. She has sparked the power within herself to do the job of making enough hormones for the rest of her life. (Please notice I said that she has helped spark her own healing ability. I am just the facilitator. With the information in this book and a healthy body, you can help yourself do the same thing.) Many Western women may find this difficult to believe, but TCM has understood the application of this natural theory as it relates to menopause for literally thousands of years.

Remember we just discussed that at the time of your first period, yang Qi is at its peak, and that when you reach the sixth cycle or age forty-two, your yin Qi takes over the controls. Now you can understand why, if a child has a problem, it is most often a yin-related issue. Here's an interesting example.

I had a young patient, Stephanie, age five, who was continually wetting her bed. Bed-wetting is almost always a problem that relates to kidney Qi deficiency. This means that the kidney's Qi is too weak or low to send the bladder the proper messages about retaining water throughout the night. However, because Stephanie was only five, and because at a young age her yang Qi should be quite high, I determined that her problem was a yin Qi deficiency. So it was my task to boost her kidney's yin Qi. The first thing I did was give her one classic herbal formula in use for centuries. The second thing I did was teach the parents how to give their daughter a moxibustion treatment. Here they learned how to heat a stick of compressed herbs and apply the heat to a special acupoint, which I showed them on Stephanie's leg. In one week, there was major improvement in her bed-wetting. After a few weeks, a problem that had gone on for several years was finally eliminated for good.

On the other hand, my patient, Gladys, seventy-two, like many women her age, also had problems holding in her urine. When an older person is incontinent, or has a urinary control issue, it usually is related to a yang Qi deficiency of the kidney. In these cases, I help the patient increase and strengthen the yang Qi of her kidney and this is what helped Gladys.

Most women who are approaching menopause and continue to age suffer from a yang Qi deficiency. So, if they can get an extra boost of yang Qi, particularly for the kidney, they have given themselves a chance at a longer life. The kidney is like an engine that supports the body's whole power system. If you can keep the power to your engine on line and strong, in other words, if you can fire up the kidney's yang Qi, you will be able to keep your body's whole system operating at a higher level for a longer time. When you do this, your body can also deal much more effectively with the root cause of the serious problems that affect many older women like osteoporosis, heart disease, breast cancer, hair loss, memory loss, skin problems, and more. And, by addressing the true source of these health problems, you can avoid the traditional Western approach of using more and more drugs to treat each successive condition as well as their side effects.

What can you do to support your kidney Qi and increase overall yang Qi or energy? Why should you do this? We'll get much deeper into this in the next chapter which covers the Five

Element Theory. Why have people the world over sought to understand this amazing blueprint?. Why does this ancient knowledge fascinate so many people? Why is it still as powerful today as it was thousands of years ago? Let's move on to the next chapter as we unravel the secrets of TCM.

TO SUMMARIZE:

- According to TCM, everything is composed of two complementary, interdependent energies: yin and yang.
- Yin and yang are never separate; one cannot exist without the other.
- Everything can be divided into yin and yang.
- Everything in the body is under the control of yin and yang energies.
- TCM uses the Theory of Yin/Yang in diagnosis and treatment.
- TCM looks at all disease or imbalances in terms of eight possible problems called the Eight Principal Syndromes: yin and yang; interior and exterior; cold and heat; deficiency and excess.
- Ideally, yin and yang should always be in harmony.
- Balance is not equal to harmony; the concept of harmony encompasses balance.
- A woman's life cycle is influenced by yin and yang energies.
- Menopausal symptoms can be categorized and treated according to the Theory of Yin/Yang.

CHAPTER 5

THE FIVE ELEMENT THEORY:
Ancient World View
of Life's Web

*T*HE Five Element Theory, like the Theory of Yin/Yang, appears deceptively simple; however, it reflects the entire Universal law in one complete, comprehensive system of related categories of things. As we've seen, ancient TCM doctors understood that all things were subject to the natural law. Today in Western society, we have almost forgotten this simple truth. Yet humankind is indeed part of nature. We are not separate or apart from it. We know it affects us, and that we affect it. I don't think anyone can doubt our effect on the earth. Look at what we've done to the environment, to the ozone layer, to the rain forests, and to our weather. Look at what we've also done to our health, and to ourselves.

Although the Five Element Theory is described in many TCM medical textbooks, most Westerners are not aware that it is also an intrinsic aspect of Chinese culture where it forms the foundation of disciplines like Feng Shui, the *I Ching,* and the martial arts. This powerful theory has gradually faded out in medical practice even in China because there are few traditional Chinese medicine doctors who can apply its deep wisdom in a practical way. The essence of the Five Element Theory has all but been lost. Part of the reason is that the ancient people who discovered this theory had a very different connection with nature than we do now. They were able to tune into things on a deep energetic level that is almost impossible to do in today's overstimulated world. They also had a profound understanding that nothing in the Universe lives a separate life. Everything is connected.

THE CONNECTEDNESS OF ALL ELEMENTS WITH THE BODY

The Five Element Theory says that everything is related to some other thing and all things are woven together into a seamless whole. If we really understood and believed this principle, we would not treat ourselves, or other people, or even our environment, the way we do. TCM practitioners learned how to apply this principle of connectedness to medical concerns thousands of years ago. Study the chart on page 68.

As you can see from the chart, there are five circles. Each of the five circles represents one of five elements: wood, fire, earth, metal, and water. Within each circle are other things that correspond with that particular element: a season, a climate or environmental factor, direction, and a color. According to TCM, all aspects of the human body and mind are also related by their nature to one of the five elements. This includes not only the principal organs—liver, heart, spleen, lung, and kidney—but every other part of the body, including emotions, and the five aspects of the soul. Therefore, within each circle is also an organ, a bowel, an emotion, a taste, a sound, and a sense organ. Before we go more deeply into this, you might want to take some time now to study this chart. The longer you study it, the more fascinating discoveries you might make. Do you see a season in which you always seem to get sick? Do you see an "opening" or tissue that always causes you health problems? Most of all, for menopausal women, do you see an emotion that particularly affects you? What organ is it connected to? If you answered anger and the liver, you are not alone. Osteoporosis is one health problem that plagues many older women. Look at the circle for the kidney. What tissue does this

CLASSIFICATION OF THINGS ACCORDING TO THE THEORY OF THE FIVE ELEMENTS

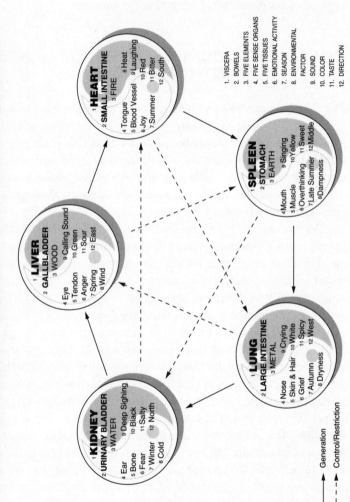

HEART
1 SMALL INTESTINE
3 FIRE
4 Tongue 8 Heat 9 Laughing
5 Blood Vessel 10 Red
6 Joy 11 Bitter
7 Summer 12 South

LIVER
2 GALLBLADDER
3 WOOD
9 Calling Sound
4 Eye 10 Green
5 Tendon 11 Sour
6 Anger 12 East
7 Spring
8 Wind

SPLEEN
2 STOMACH
3 EARTH
9 Singing 10 Yellow
4 Mouth 11 Sweet
5 Muscle 12 Middle
6 Overthinking
7 Late Summer
8 Dampness

KIDNEY
2 URINARY BLADDER
3 WATER
9 Deep Sighing
4 Ear 10 Black
5 Bone 11 Salty
6 Fear 12 North
7 Winter
8 Cold

LUNG
1 LARGE INTESTINE
3 METAL
9 Crying
4 Nose 10 White
5 Skin & Hair 11 Spicy
6 Grief 12 West
7 Autumn
8 Dryness

1. VISCERA
2. BOWELS
3. FIVE ELEMENTS
4. FIVE SENSE ORGANS
5. FIVE TISSUES
6. EMOTIONAL ACTIVITY
7. SEASON
8. ENVIRONMENTAL FACTOR
9. SOUND
10. COLOR
11. TASTE
12. DIRECTION

→ Generation
- - → Control/Restriction

organ relate to? You can see that it's the bone. That's why TCM treats osteoporosis by treating the kidney. You can also understand why taking large quantities of calcium, while it may help, cannot, by itself, address the root cause of this condition.

RELATIONSHIPS OF GENERATION AND CONTROL

The Five Element Theory is one of the oldest theories of how the Universe operates. It was adapted by the ancient TCM doctors and used to help them in their medical practice. As you can see, each of the five elements has its own individual system relating to eleven categories of things, but all of these elemental systems have an inseparable connection to each other. For the whole system to function in harmony, two dynamic relationships of generation and control must operate smoothly. To use the Five Element Theory in diagnosis and treatment, TCM analyzes these dynamic relationships of the elements and therefore their circles. It is vitally interested in aspects of generation and control between the organs.

It is important to understand that the Five Elements themselves are also not inert substances. They are fundamental energies in nature, and they too, like yin and yang, are continually in motion. Each element generates or gives birth to another. In TCM, these element pairs are known as mother and child.

Each element also restrains or controls another. The right amount of control keeps all the elements in proper proportion and balance. This kind of interaction enables all the elements—and all the other related aspects of the organ listed in each circle—to work as one harmonious system. From the health perspective, if these relationships are balanced, you are feeling well and strong; if any of the relationships become unbalanced, you will suffer from various discomforts and health problems.

From the spiritual perspective, if you can maintain harmony among the five emotions of the five major organs, then you will remain unaffected by external or internal change. If you reach this stage, stress, which occurs when outside events affect your emotions, cannot bother you anymore. Depression wouldn't bother you either because you would not be attached to emotions that occur in your daily life. (You would experience the emotions, but you would not be engaged with or attached to them.) Antidepressants would become unnecessary. You wouldn't get mad at things that happen, or at things that someone does to you. You wouldn't be excessively happy (even if you won the lottery!). You wouldn't be concerned with passing judgment on the things that happen in your life, or to other people. Material and visible things would become unimportant and eventually meaningless. This produces a true state of spirituality.

Let's explore the elemental circles together so you can understand what I mean. Start with the circle that contains the element water. TCM identifies water as the mother (or the generator because it takes water to nourish the trees) of wood (likewise wood is the child of water, its mother). Now, follow the dotted arrow from the water circle. You can see that water also has another job or function. It controls the element of fire (of course that makes sense, because naturally water puts out fire). If we start at the circle that contains the element wood, you can see that it is the mother of fire.

Following the dotted arrow across, you can see that wood controls the earth. Take the time to look at all the circles and identify the patterns of connections. Understanding the Five Element Theory will give you more insight to understanding perimenopause or menopause. It will also help you later when we talk about the organs, their relationships and lifestyle habits that you can change that will allow you to make a smooth transition through menopause without hormones.

Now we can take the Five Element Theory one step further as we look at the whole human body. As I said before, all aspects of the human body and mind are also related by their nature to one of the five elements. So if we again look at the circle with the element of water, we find the kidney there. Following the same pattern as above, you can see that the kidney is the mother of the liver (the liver, then, is the child of the kidney). This is nature's pattern of generation between these two organs. If we follow the dotted arrow from the circle with the element of water, you can see that the Qi of the kidney exerts control over, or keeps in balance, the Qi of the heart.

Following this ancient blueprint, here's what we find:

MOTHER AND CHILD RELATIONSHIPS

- The kidney is mother of the liver.
- The liver is mother of the heart.
- The heart is mother of the spleen.
- The spleen is mother of the lung.
- The lung is mother of the kidney.

CONTROL RELATIONSHIPS

- The kidney controls the heart.
- The liver controls the spleen.
- The heart controls the lung.
- The spleen controls the kidney.
- The lung controls the liver.

Now that you understand which are the mother organs and which are the children organs and which organs control the other, you're probably wondering what this framework means and how it applies to health and the transition of menopause. Here's why this information is so vital. Without the function of control, generation would be excessive or too much. This relationship operates just like a real mother and child. Unless the mother puts certain limits on her child, for example, she or he would be totally wild and out of control! I think you can begin to see and appreciate what this means. I also want to emphasize that this is not an abstract concept. This is the way your body operates in reality. When I relate these things, so many of my patients exclaim, "I never heard that." Or, "I wish I had understood these things a long time ago."

But the truth is there was no way for them as individuals brought up in a Western culture, to have this knowledge. Our meeting is called fate. Chinese philosophy would call writing this book and sharing this ancient wisdom about menopause fate. Likewise, your reading this information is also fate.

The functions of generation and control enable all the organs—and all the elements—to work in harmony. If their relationship is good, you are healthy. If any of the relationships among the organs is not good, if it is "broken," you will have a problem. In order to have good digestion, for example, the liver must exert the right amount of control on the stomach. Too much or too little control both cause problems. You may suffer from abdominal distention or indigestion; you may burp a lot and have a sour taste in your mouth (the taste associated with the liver). Or you might start gaining weight. What appears to be a stomach problem is really a condition being generated by a liver function disorder. Simply put, the liver isn't working the way it should. Efforts to fix the stomach can offer only limited relief.

When I work with patients who have these kinds of problems, before I educate them about TCM, they say, "I've been through all the Western medical tests you can imagine and I can tell you that my liver is perfect!" I tell them to be careful. "The scientific tests of your physical liver may be normal, because your problem is still at the function stage. Modern science and modern medicine have no way to measure organ function or the amount of Qi you have." I also tell them, "Think about your headache; two years ago you didn't have this problem and now you're suffering from these headaches all the time. You've changed your job, and you've taken many drugs and nothing's really relieved it. I think you know you have a problem, even if all your medical tests are normal. Your condition is not yet within the range of Western medical tests. By the time it is, it will have progressed to a much more serious condition. Treat it now. Don't wait until later." Here's a good example.

My patient Suzanne, age forty-nine, came to me complaining that she had had a migraine headache almost daily for more than six months. Naturally, she had seen many doctors and had tried many different prescriptions. She had even had an MRI and a CT scan. All her tests were normal. She told me she was scared because her tests showed nothing, but she was feeling terrible and had never had this kind of severe headache for such a long time before. When we discussed her period, she told me that for the past two years it had become increasingly irregular. At first, this migraine came right before her period. For the past few months though, her migraine headache had come more often. I checked her pulses and found that her liver pulse had a very thready and sluggish beat. From her pulse diagnosis and her other physical conditions I knew her migraine headache was caused by a liver function disorder and a kidney Qi deficiency. Using the Five Element Theory, we can see that this is a mother-child problem. To fix it, I needed to help her make her liver function more smoothly again and to help her increase kidney Qi.

So, I gave her acupuncture and a TCM herbal formula. After two treatments, Suzanne told me that her migraine headaches had stopped. This case study helps us understand that function problems can cause very real discomfort and that they are not in the patient's head, they are just beyond the ability of scientific medical tests to perceive. If you're like Suzanne, keep trying to find someone who will help you identify the root cause of your problem. Do not try to cover it up or mask the symptoms. While I don't object to people trying to obtain relief from their pain or discomfort, I always urge them not to stop there.

Applying the Five Element Theory to Real-Life Problems

Earlier we talked about the importance of the kidney with its Inborn Qi as an important source of support for all the organs. Strong kidney Qi is absolutely critical to support its child, the liver, and to control or restrain the fire of the heart. Remember when most Western women reach menopausal age, their kidney Qi is already in a weakened state and their liver is usually functioning poorly. Like any child, the liver, whose energy is low due to the stresses of daily life, "sucks" or "takes" the Qi it needs from its mother, the kidney. And like most children, the liver always wants more, and like a good and giving mother, the kidney is there to oblige. Unfortunately, the child's constant need for additional Qi can take its toll on the mother. This is when problems arise in the function of the kidney too.

One of my patients, Angela, age fifty-five, came to see me with heart palpitations, sleeping problems, and heartburn. As we just saw, the Qi of the kidney should exert the proper amount of control over the Qi of the heart. I could tell from her symptoms and a pulse diagnosis that her kidney Qi was too weak to "put out the fire" of her heart. So I treated her kidney with great success. If I had just treated her heart, we might have been able to decrease some of her symptoms, but the underlying problem would have remained, and might have progressed.

Another patient, Patricia, age fifty-seven, was experiencing night sweats. She said she often had a dry cough, chest pains, and shortness of breath. When I examined her I saw that she had dry skin, a problem she said she had had for as long as she could remember. Given her age and symptoms, I knew right away that Patricia had a kidney Qi deficiency. But what was the cause? In her case, it was *not* the liver: it was her lung. How did I come to that conclusion? If you look at the Five Element chart, you can see that the skin is the "opening" to the outside world of the lung; skin problems are, generally speaking, related to the lung and its companion organ the large intestine. So Patricia's long time dry skin condition was a major clue, as was the dry cough that she was experiencing nightly, to the true source of her problems.

Many organs can cause a cough, but when a person also has dry skin, the problem almost always originates in the lung. So why was Patricia's lung problem also a kidney problem? Look at the Five Element Theory chart again. The lung is the mother of the kidney, and for whatever reason, Patricia's lung, the mother organ, did not have enough Qi to support its child—the kidney. To help her get relief rapidly, I treated both organs at the same time. The treatment for her lung, however, was not just directed at soothing her dry cough, but also at boosting lung Qi and kidney Qi, as well. Given her age and the uncomfortable night sweats she was also experiencing, I treated Patricia's liver function disorder too. Remember, the reason for boosting Patricia's lung and kidney Qi was to bring her organs back up to full power so she could heal herself.

The Five Element Theory is a very powerful technique when used correctly and with intuition. It can provide great insights into the source of a wide variety of diseases and illnesses. In Patricia's case, I applied the theory of the mother/child relationship. However, with other people, I apply the theory of the control relationship.

Another patient, Jewell, age forty-six, came to see me regularly. She was overweight and had poor digestion, stomach distention, and loose stool. Jewell also couldn't eat cold things such as dairy products, had frequent nighttime urination, and hot flashes. In addition, her tongue had a thick, white coating. In Jewell's case, she had a lot of problems related to the stomach. Now remember in the Five Element Theory chart, the earth (the spleen/stomach) controls water (the kidney). When the earth does not perform properly or exhibit its normal properties, it cannot absorb water, and there is too much of it with nowhere to go (like when there is a flood). Jewell had come to me with a serious dampness problem, which TCM recognizes as a kidney problem. The true source of her discomfort was that her stomach Qi could not control her kidney Qi. It was not strong enough to keep their relationship balanced and harmonious. These two organs had stopped communicating well with each other. Her white tongue reflected a common symptom of stomach dampness. (This is something you can easily check for yourself.) To fix her root condition, I treated both organs.

APPLYING THE FIVE ELEMENT THEORY TO EMOTIONAL PROBLEMS

We've seen how the Five Element Theory works with organ relationships, now let's examine how this complex TCM theory works with emotional connections. As we've seen, each elemental circle also has its own associated emotion. Studying the Five Element Theory chart is like studying a blueprint for the body's systems. You can gain a lot of insight into how one organ's problem can affect so many organs. Or how a problem with one of the body's tissues connects with an organ.

For example, one of the major problems after menopause is osteoporosis, which is a loss of bone density. Many women take calcium supplements or even estrogen to prevent this problem. The Five Element Theory chart, however, points us to the root cause of osteoporosis. The bone is the tissue of the kidney. As I've said, TCM believes that to really prevent bone loss, you must first treat the kidney. And, the Five Element Theory chart also tells us that the kidney controls the heart. If you have a kidney Qi deficiency, then you might unbalance the relationship between your kidney and your heart. This can cause heart disease. The more you study the Five Element Theory chart, the more you can apply the understanding of how fundamental underlying relationships must work properly to keep your body functioning in harmony.

ELEMENTS, ORGANS, EMOTIONS

- Water (the kidney) is fear
- Wood (the liver) is anger
- Fire (the heart) is joy
- Earth (the spleen) is overthinking or worrying
- Metal (the lung) is sadness

As many women reach menopausal age, there are numerous emotional challenges in their lives. Today's woman is often expected to be everything to everyone. This kind of pressure and responsibility is tremendous and takes a very real toll on women's health. Often, the years right before and during menopause represent a time for major changes in a woman's life—including divorce or leaving a partner after many years; children leaving home for good; parents dying; loss of friends through illness or moves; transitions in job responsibilities, health declines, and more.

TCM understands that an excess of different emotions can be pathogenic in nature and cause the function of different organs to fall out of balance. If an illness is diagnosed as having its root cause in an unbalanced emotion, TCM says—as you may recall from the Introduction—that the best way to treat it is to counter it with its controlling emotion. In this situation, it is most common for emotional causes to be related to the function of control—generally speaking a lack of control. Here the Five Element Theory is a superb and accurate guide.

To begin to really understand the correspondences or relationships between things, it is helpful to again study the Five Element Theory chart. Look at the individual circles once more. In the circle relating to the liver, for example, you can see that the associated emotion is anger. (Remember that the liver is the most important organ for women's health.) Following the arrows, you can see that the lung controls the liver; at the emotional energy level, sadness controls anger. Anger controls overthinking. Overthinking controls fear. Fear controls happiness. And happiness controls sadness.

Here are some interesting examples of how TCM's ancient masters applied the Five Element Theory to treat health conditions stemming from emotional causes.

SHOCK FIXES EXCESS HAPPINESS

In Chinese culture as in many others, having a male child is extremely important. One old woman worried constantly about her son who had three daughters, but no male children. She worried about her family's ancestors and how the line would not continue without a male. She constantly prayed and made offerings at a nearby shrine for a male child. One day, her son told her that his wife was pregnant again. During her daughter-in-law's pregnancy, the old woman prayed deeply for a grandson. When she heard that her grandchild was a male, she became elated—so happy that her line would continue. Her happiness was unbounded. It literally exploded within her. All of a sudden, the old woman lost all her strength; she became listless, and could not walk any great length or at a reasonable pace. Her son became alarmed and brought her to many different doctors and acupuncturists.

One day they visited a new doctor. The son went in first to explain his mother's condition and when it first started. The minute the doctor saw the old woman, he picked up a medical instrument and rushed toward her with great urgency saying "Your son has told me how serious your problem is. We must do surgery on your knees right away. Please come with me at once!" The old woman looked at him in absolute fright for a split second, then ran from the office as fast as she could. Her problem went away and her ability to walk returned. Because he understood that the root cause of the physical problem was an emotional one, this ancient doctor was able to use happiness' controlling emotion of fear to fix the problem.

OVERTHINKING CREATES PHYSICAL REALITY

Once there was a woman who had a nightmare during which she saw herself drink a bowl of soup with a snake in it. The next morning she woke up with a terrible stomachache convinced that the snake was actually inside her. After that, she often had very bad stomachaches that no one could fix. Eventually this discomfort would not leave her. No matter what the treatment, she remained the same. She began to lose weight and weaken. Her husband became very worried about his wife and asked one special doctor for help. After much discussion with the husband, the doctor understood that the true source of the woman's problem was her bad dream. The doctor told her husband that to relieve this kind of problem they had to make her believe that the snake had left her body. He told the man to buy a small snake and put it inside their toilet first. Then, the doctor told the woman: "Don't worry. I can fix your problem. I have a special herb that can kill your snake and cause it to leave your body." He told the woman to drink his herbal concoction and remain in a dark room with incense where the toilet was in a dark corner. About a half an hour later, the woman had diarrhea and went to the toilet. Later, her housekeeper rushed in to say that she had passed a snake. After this event, the woman never had a stomach problem again.

USING EMOTIONAL QI TO HEAL PHYSICAL PROBLEMS

While emotions can often cause problems, such as when you hear about a friend's death and cry uncontrollably, or you're fired and suddenly become exhausted, they can also cure certain conditions. Here's one interesting story.

In ancient times, a woman developed a problem with her arm. It seemed she couldn't unbend it and drop it down by her side. She suffered from this condition for quite a while, but could not find anyone to help her. One day she heard about a doctor in the neighboring town. She made the journey with her husband and children to his office and during her first visit explained to him that she could not remember how this condition started, but that she had no problem with her bones or her muscles. It was a mystery to her. After the doctor heard this, he examined her arms very carefully. Then he said to her: "I must treat this by putting acupuncture needles along the inside of your leg. I think this is the best way and you must undress right now and take off your trousers." At the same time, the doctor moved forward and motioned as if he was going to remove her pants in front of all the people in his office. The woman instinctively reached down to grab her pants with her bad arm. After that, the doctor explained that he was actually trying to stimulate her own healing power to relieve her long-time physical problem. This story helps illustrate that the body has a memory of its own. The doctor recognized what many modern people fail to understand—often emotions can remain locked in the body and can look like physical problems. Most people don't recognize that chronic unbalanced emotions cause physical problems, When the physical part of the problem manifests itself, it's usually very deeply ingrained in the body and our attention goes naturally enough to the visible, not the invisible. It takes a skilled doctor to probe for this kind of information and understand how to release long-held emotions that are creating physical problems.

And now, here are some modern-day examples of this technique.

SADNESS RELIEVES ANGER

My patient Shirley, age forty-five, was divorced. She hated her job and from what I could tell, carried a great deal of anger inside her. I could see that she had a liver function problem (anger being the emotion related to the liver). Which organ controls the liver? The lung. The emotion related to the lung is sadness. So I told Shirley to go see a movie with a really sad ending. "It'll make you cry," I told her, "and after you cry, you won't feel this chronic weight of anger anymore." If you refer back to the Five Element Chart, you'll see that the lung's emotion of sadness can relieve or control the liver's emotion of anger. I must admit she looked at me a little strangely, but she really wanted to get better and, lucky for me, she trusted me. So that's exactly what she did. She was amazed to find that this simple, easy treatment actually worked and she did indeed manage to gain almost immediate relief from her anger and feel better. This also helped her liver function begin to improve. With additional treatment with herbs and acupuncture, her entrance into menopause became a smooth and healthy one.

Here's another true story. Mary worried constantly. She was always thinking, thinking, thinking. According to the Five Element Theory, overthinking is associated with the stomach. So I tried to help her by letting her experience anger. (The liver's emotion can control that of the spleen's.)

Mary was always calling my office, worried about different health problems, especially her lack of appetite. So for a short time, I told my clinic's doctor to help her, but tell her I was not available. Not being able to talk to me directly made her very angry. After a week or two of not being able to communicate, Mary came to my office and quite angrily told me that I was wrong for not calling her back. The very next day she came to see me and apologized for being so angry, and she wanted me to know that she was feeling much better and, to her utter surprise, her appetite had returned. That's when I told her that I wanted to find a way to help her relieve her overthinking. In my opinion, this was the best way to deal with the root cause of her problem. Without understanding that the source of her stomach problem was an emotional one, Mary could have spent years looking for help and might never have resolved her health condition.

EMOTIONAL PROBLEMS CAN CAUSE PHYSICAL PROBLEMS

Chinese doctors were using psychology hundreds of years before their counterparts in the West. Many centuries of experience have taught us that emotional problems can indeed cause physical ones—such as the toll stress and anger take on peoples' lives and livers.

For example, I've noticed that a large number of my Western women patients complain of chronic postnasal drip that seems to be accompanied by a small lump in their throat. They usually blame their condition on sinus problems. The lump, however, is a very interesting one. They cannot swallow this lump, nor can they spit it out. Some have even gone as far as having an operation on their nose. According to classical Chinese medicine, this is a physical condition with an emotional cause. So common is this condition, that ancient doctors even had a name for it—*mei he qi.* Literally, these women have a lump of Qi stuck in their throat. To fix this, the doctor must rebalance the liver's function.

From my experience treating this condition, the best way to deal with it is to first help the patient recognize that her physical condition is caused by her emotions. Then I add acupuncture and herbs. But, often this problem is caused by a very deep anger and sadness, with which the woman has not yet dealt. Once she understands that the root cause of this problem is emotional, then she has to be willing to let her anger or sadness go. If she cannot do this, the best that I can do is treat her symptoms. Sooner or later any similar emotions will trigger the same problem. No amount of medication or medical procedures for this kind of post-nasal drip will ever solve this condition. Addressing the root cause is what counts. My patients are so smart. Once they begin to understand how their bodies work, they are really good about taking responsibility for their own healing.

Here's another example.

Janice, age fifty-two, came to see me because she had suffered from a stabbing pain behind her eyes for six months. Nothing could relieve it. Pain medication didn't help, and now she was thinking about going to see a psychiatrist. Then I examined her pulse, and said, "No, there's something wrong with your liver function." I asked her if there was something that was upsetting her or that had caused her to become excessively angry about six months ago when her eye pain began. She thought back and said yes. "That's when my husband and I started getting a divorce." I told her "Yes, your pain is really coming from anger, which has caused your liver Qi to stagnate." She loved her husband very much and she was very lonely and sad. Although she thought she had resolved her angry feelings, the energy of them had remained stuck inside.

I asked her how she commuted to New York City every day. She said by train. I asked who sat next to her, men or women? She said mostly men, sometimes women. I said, "Okay, you come into New York and sit on the train for forty minutes every day and what do you do?" She said that she usually slept. So I teased her, "Look at you. Almost every day you get to sleep with a different man!" Then, using what my master has taught me about Chinese psychology, I said, "When you get to New York City, everybody gets off the train and goes to their own destinations. Think about it, your life is like this train. For decades, you and your husband were passengers on the same train. But he had to get off and now you have to continue. You are born here not just for your husband. You are born here for you. Together you traveled on the same train for a certain amount of time, but you must continue your mission, you must continue with your life, just as he has to continue with his mission and his life. If you really want to heal your eye pain for good, you must let go of your anger. Remember that the eye is the 'opening' to the outside world for your liver. You should do this to heal your liver."

After we talked, Janice said that she never thought of her life this way. She left with a new viewpoint and renewed hope and recognition that her life had meaning beyond her current pain and sorrow. She left with the will to get over her anger and hurt. I tried to help her by showing her a different way to look at this situation. Life at this point had to change for her. It's not that her husband was wrong or that he was a bad person; it's that she had to let her anger go and make positive changes to keep herself healthy.

Here's an ancient story about the concept of letting go that you might find helpful.

As a Buddhist master and his student were walking toward the riverbank, they suddenly saw a young woman who was very distressed. This was somewhat of a problem because in their religion they were forbidden to look at, or even speak with, a woman. She, however, was deeply upset because she had to cross this river in order to continue her journey to reach her sick father. She begged the master and his student to help her get across the river. Very gently, the master picked her up and carried her across the river, then put her down on the other side, said goodbye, and went on his way with the student.

Because he was a master, he could tell that his student was quite upset, even though the student was silent for the rest of their journey. Finally, that night as they were preparing for bed, he said to his student, "Is everything all right?" "No!" the student exploded. "Everything is not all right. You spoke with a woman today and then carried her across the river. How could you do that? Our religion tell us that this is wrong." The monk replied, "Really, when did I do this?" "This morning, this morning!!" his student shouted, becoming more agitated. "Oh, this morning. Now I remember," said the master, "I already put her down. Now tell me, why you have been carrying her all day long?"

One of the most comprehensive self-diagnosis tools I can offer you is the Five Element Theory Chart. I recommend you spend time studying this so you can understand the critical role balanced emotions play in remaining strong and healthy. This is particularly important for women during menopause. If you become ill, you can ask yourself: "Was I angry first, and then became ill?" Or, "Did I become ill first and then become angry?" Remember excess anger can damage your liver function, but it is also important to remember that liver damage can likewise change your personality and make you testy and angry.

Now that you understand the main theories of TCM, let's go on to discover how each of the five major organs and their partner organs work in greater detail. This information and the stories of my patients should give you more insight into how to remain healthy through menopause and beyond.

TO SUMMARIZE:
- TCM divides all things into five elements: water, wood, fire, earth, and metal.
- Each of these five elements also corresponds with a viscera or major organ, a bowel, or partner organ, sense organ, body tissue, emotion, season, environmental factor, sound, color, taste, and direction.

- In TCM, the five major organ systems have two essential connections: generation (one is the mother and child of another) and control (one keeps another in balance).
- TCM applies the Five Element Theory to physical problems.
- TCM applies the Five Element Theory to emotional problems.

CHAPTER 6

BALANCING YOUR ORGANS' RELATIONSHIPS FOR A HORMONE-FREE TRANSITION

*B*EFORE we begin this chapter, I'd like to remind you that when TCM talks about an organ, its definition is broader than that of Western medicine. When TCM refers to an organ, it is not only discussing the physical structure, but a whole complex of functions both physiological and psychological. (That is why TCM refers to the lung and kidney in the singular to distinguish their meaning from the physical organs themselves.)

As we've just seen, the Five Element Theory shows us that, besides its function in the various systems of the body, each organ also governs a body tissue, sometimes called "sinew," and a sense organ (the organ's "opening" such as the eye or ear), is related to a particular emotion, and houses one of the five aspects of the soul. Each organ also has a partner organ. All of these relationships are under the dynamics of generation and control. By now, I think you can appreciate how complex your body is.

PARTNER ORGANS

- Kidney and bladder
- Liver and gallbladder
- Heart and small intestine

- Spleen and stomach
- Lung and large intestine

All of the functions, or jobs, of the organs are closely inter-related and can have a strong effect on one another. For instance, each organ, as I explained in Chapter 4, is especially susceptible to its corresponding emotion. Here again we can see the Yin/Yang Theory at work. For example, all the major organs are viscera and considered yin organs. Their partner organs are bowels and are considered yang organs. We've also seen that when one organ has a problem, so, to some degree, will its partner organ. Because of the connections they share through Qi, TCM understands that you can treat the major organ by treating its partner. For example, if you have constipation, which is related to the large intestine, you might try one of many Western remedies for adding roughage or flaxseed. TCM knows that it can treat the large intestine through its partner organ the lung and still relieve the constipation.

We are very conditioned in Western culture to view our body as separate parts with no relationship or connection with another. When you think about this, it's almost shocking to see how naïve it is to believe that when we hurt in one place our body doesn't experience or feel it in other areas as well. Think of modern advertising: take a pill for this headache; take a pill for that stomachache; drink this tea for that fever; use this nasal spray for that sinus condition. Because we don't have a framework of understanding about how the body is connected, we obey these commands without comprehending what *other* body parts we're affecting, and in some cases damaging. It is my hope that the following knowledge about the organs and their relationships will provide new insight into the way your body really operates. It will, I believe, help you reach a much deeper level of understanding of menopause and the control you have to treat it naturally without hormones.

While your organs have several physical connections with each other, the most important connection, according to TCM, is their energetic or Qi connection. This Qi relationship can be direct or indirect. Organs that have no physical connection with each other, for instance your lung and large intestine, actually share a very important energy connection through their meridians. Your lung also has an important energy connection with its "child," the kidney and with the liver, the organ that it controls. Western medicine tends to see only the physical, scientific relationships among your body's organs. TCM's ancient medical framework goes beyond the physical and maps out your body's inherent Qi-based connections. From this understanding it is possible to develop diagnoses of the root cause of a health condition.

The good news is that both Western and Chinese medical systems are moving toward each other in interesting ways. Western medicine, for example, has now learned that your stomach is related to your brain. Recent research has uncovered the way epithelial cells in the stomach's lining communicate with the brain—a scientific window on "gut feelings." Western researchers now know the stomach can have a powerful effect on what goes on in the brain.

TCM has understood the energy connection between the brain and the stomach for thousands of years. Follow the Five Element Theory: the stomach is considered the "child" of the heart. In TCM, the heart is the organ that controls all mental activities. The skillful TCM doctor often treats mental problems by also treating the stomach—this would be called a classical example of healing the "child" through its "mother." Though they've arrived at the same understanding, TCM uses Qi to understand the human body; Western medicine works within the physical paradigm.

Here's an analogy that might help you understand this kind of mother/child relationship in the Five Element Theory better. If your children have problems at school, either related to studying or their relationships with other children, the principal will call you, as the parent, to come in and talk things over. Although they may speak with your child directly, they know that the problem will only really get solved by involving you.

So now let's delve deeply into the organs and see how their relationships affect menopause.

THE LIVER

The Liver and the Flow of Qi

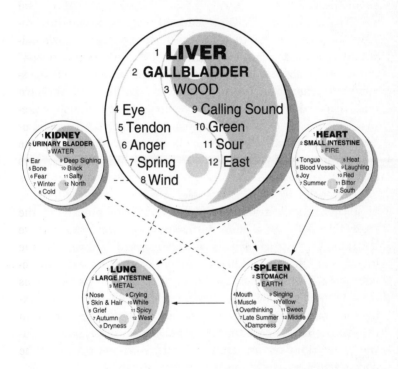

As I've emphasized a number of times throughout this book, all women's health problems—either directly or indirectly—relate to liver function. We've also said that classical TCM theory states that the liver is the most important organ for women's health. As long as you can keep your liver Qi flowing smoothly and the liver itself functioning in harmony with its four other major partner organs, you can enjoy good health.

In the Five Element Theory, the liver's partner organ is the gallbladder. Its element is wood. The opening gate to the outside of the body is the eye. The tissue it controls is the tendon. The emotion that can affect the liver is anger. The seasonal energy and time which matches the liver's is spring. Its environmental factor is wind. The color related to liver energy is green. The taste that goes directly to the liver is sour. The direction or location is East.

The nature of liver Qi is reflected in its corresponding element of wood: like the roots of a tree, liver Qi likes to move outward freely and to reach everywhere. TCM thinks of this "wood" mostly as bamboo, a long, flexible reed that adapts to changing conditions. The liver governs the flow of Qi or life force throughout the body. It also smoothes and regulates the circulation of that inseparable pair: Qi and blood. Remember, the *Nei Jing* tells us that the liver is "the root of stopping all extremes," so that if the flow of Qi or blood becomes blocked or stuck, it is your liver's job to free it.

According to TCM, any problem that occurs on the left side of your body indicates a liver dysfunction. (Any problem on the right side indicates a lung dysfunction.) If you always get a headache on your left side, or your left nostril is always stuffed up, or your left shoulder has a pain, or you notice a weakness in your left ankle, or you always fall on your left side or bump into something on your left side, then you should recognize that your liver is not working properly. Even if all scientific tests are normal, you definitely need to work at healing your liver because the way its working or functioning is "off." A knowledgeable TCM doctor would recognize this problem immediately.

Your liver has an important relationship with your spleen, particularly because they share responsibility for maintaining good digestion. If your spleen does not get the proper support from your liver, it will not be able to transform food into the life-sustaining elements of Qi and blood. Your liver, which stores your blood, depends in turn upon your spleen to provide an adequate supply of nutrition. Remember, deficient liver blood shows up especially in those areas of the body that correspond with the liver's element of wood: your nails, eyes, ligaments, and tendons.

Here's an example that is similar to Janice's in the previous chapter: One day, an attractive businesswoman Sally, in her mid-thirties and in pretty good health, came to my office complaining that her left eye had been burning and hurting for about six months. She had tried many over-the-counter remedies and had seen several ophthalmologists, but her problem persisted. Her pulse diagnosis told me that her condition was being caused by liver Qi stagnation. In the "asking" part of my examination, I inquired about her daily life. I asked her whether she had experienced anything sad or distressing six months ago around the time her problem began.

She told me that just about that time she had gone through a very difficult divorce that produced tremendous anger and resentment in her. She felt, however, that she had dealt with it and had put her emotions to rest. At that point, I identified that the source of her eye problem was coming from an excess of liver heat, and was able to work out a treatment plan with her that included acupuncture and herbs. We also talked deeply about the fact that the root cause of her physical problem was her excessive and unrelieved anger. To fix her problem, we then discussed a number of ways that would help her let this anger go, including three very simple, time-tested TCM ways to release anger:

- Break several glass bottles (in an enclosed area with no one around);
- Throw a dozen eggs;
- Scream as loud as you can. (This one works especially well when you're in the car.)

You may think these are pretty simple, low-tech ways to get rid of anger, but I can tell you from an energy standpoint, they can do the trick. Why? Because you cause something to break and dissipate or relieve itself, in this case it is the energy of the anger that is held inside. Some of my patients ask me about using a punching bag, and I warn them not to do that. I tell them: "Remember your physics, if you punch with all your might and generate a certain kind of force, what happens? An equal force is returned to you! Remember you want to relieve and get rid of the anger, not have it smack you back." The three ways mentioned above have been used (and prescribed, I might add) for centuries in TCM. And, believe it or not, they do work! Once you do it, I think you'll love the feeling you get. In fact, many of my patients come back and say: "Why didn't you tell me to buy two dozen eggs?" The feeling they get from releasing this energy is very healing. So what if your family and your neighbors think you're a little strange.

So, Sally also worked at getting rid of her anger, not suppressing or internalizing it. Within three weekly visits, her pain had virtually disappeared. Although her symptoms were alleviated, I told her that she could only heal completely if she worked at rebalancing her liver's Qi with certain foods and lifestyle changes. Above all, she had to find a way to let her negative emotions go. Sally really wanted to get completely better, so she made a number of changes that over time healed her problem.

Liver and Blood: One of the Most Important Partnerships for Women's Health

The liver's role with regard to blood is especially important for women. A properly functioning menstrual cycle depends upon the liver to regulate the flow of blood (as well as store it). If your liver Qi becomes unbalanced—either too much, what TCM terms excessive, or too little, which it terms deficient—symptoms like PMS, irregular periods, headaches, cramps, and distending pain in the breasts will occur on a regular basis.

In the West, most of us would not automatically think to connect these symptoms with the liver. Yet, such problems are the norm for many women who suffer through difficult menstrual cycles year after year. They don't realize that these debilitating conditions are symptomatic of a deeper internal imbalance that their own bodies can resolve, given the proper support. It's important to recognize that these are internal warning signs for problems that may appear later on, including uncomfortable menopausal symptoms, or even breast or uterine cancer.

Once again, I am amazed by the number of my patients who tell me that they have routinely taken painkillers monthly for years, sometimes, decades, because they believe "that's just the way things are with women's menstrual problems." I try to get them to understand, as I hope you will, that this is not normal. I really want to emphasize this point: A healthy body does not have monthly menstrual problems, no matter how many scientific tests say you are well.

If you are menopausal or postmenopausal, a smoothly functioning liver is essential to good health. Even after your period stops, the proper circulation of Qi and blood is still a vital process that must continue for a woman to remain in good health. Since the liver's function is sensitive to so many energy changes (like seasons, emotions, weather, and the like) and is related to so many organs, managing emotions to keep liver Qi flowing smoothly is crucial for women of all ages in the prevention of breast masses and cancer.

The Liver, Unbalanced Emotions, and Stress

TCM views the high incidence of breast cancer in Western society as liver Qi stagnation caused by prolonged stress and emotional excess—especially anger and overthinking. Just as your liver's job is to keep the flow of Qi and blood running smoothly, it also must keep your emotions flowing evenly as well. Poor liver function can show up in its corresponding emotions of anger, rage, depression, and stress, or in a more general feeling of uneven moods, like frustration, irritability, or nervous tension.

If you suffer from a liver function imbalance, you might feel frustrated easily and your emotions may tend to get blocked and stuck. You might have trouble unwinding from the day's tensions. You may also have difficulty in letting things go. You may use your Qi and emotions to dwell on the same issues or problems over and over. Some of the things you think about may have occurred long ago in the past, but you still let them consume your precious Qi or vital energy in the present.

While poor organ function can cause emotional problems, the reverse is more often the case. Likewise, a poorly functioning liver can have a profound effect on your whole body—especially in relationship to the organs with which it shares important partnerships like the stomach or the heart. It is impossible to overstate the importance of reducing stress in your life. Stress is a kind of energy or vibration that goes right to your liver where it can either cause or aggravate many problems: from migraine headaches to high blood pressure, to insomnia, to menstrual and digestive problems. Stress is more than a daily annoyance or burden. According to TCM, it can create the root cause of life-threatening conditions.

During the fourteenth century, a very famous Chinese physician, Dr. Dan Qi Zhu (A.D. 1281–1358), based his own theories on the work of the *Nei Jing*. His *Dan Qi Xin Fa* discusses breast cancer this way: "Because the wife does not enjoy a good relationship with her husband, nor does she enjoy good relationships with family members and others, then chronic anger, depression, worry, and nervousness will accumulate in her day by day. This condition, if left unchecked, will cause a spleen Qi or 'digestive system' disorder, as well as liver Qi stagnation. Eventually, this will cause a small lump within the breast that causes no pain and no itchiness. Many years later, this lump will turn into a different shape (much like a craggy rock with many holes), which is called 'yan,' or cancer. If the lump takes on this shape, it is very difficult to fix." Before Christopher Columbus had discovered the New World, TCM doctors understood the root cause of breast cancer and called this condition by name.

So you see, when Qi or energy stagnates in the meridians over time, a small seed can progress to a cancerous mass. Energy literally becomes transformed into matter. Then, the five major organs begin to spiral out of balance. When Qi does not flow freely through the meridians and the organs have fallen out of balance, the body is too weak to defend itself from internal and external pathogens.

Uterine cancer also relates to your liver. Everything having to do with the uterus depends upon the healthy function of the liver and proper flow of its Qi. Stagnant Qi and blood due to poor liver function can cause the formation of hard lumps, masses, and tumors, such as uterine fibroids and ovarian cysts. If prolonged and severe enough, Qi stagnation or the blockage of Qi can lead to cancer. So it's vital that you take care of yourself today and every day. Don't wait until you feel terrible to get help. Don't tell yourself: "I'm not *that* sick." The time to prevent illness or disease is when your Qi is strong enough to fend them off. I also want you to remember that when it comes to staying healthy, there are no "quick fixes." Good health is built minute by minute, hour by hour, and day by day. I am not talking about drudgery here. I am talking about a joyful process of understanding that you have a unique place in the world and a unique mission you were born to accomplish. Having optimum health can make your spiritual journey a deeply rewarding one.

TCM'S TOP TEN CONDITIONS THAT INDICATE A LIVER DYSFUNCTION

1. Menstrual cycle problems: PMS, cramps, breast tenderness
2. Yeast infections.
3. Anger
4. Mood swings and irritability
5. Brittle nails
6. Headaches on either side of the head
7. Eye irritation
8. Tendon problems
9. Stress
10. Bloating and indigestion

THE HEART: KING OF THE ORGANS

In TCM, the heart is considered the king of all the organs. Ancient texts say that "if the king is happy, there is peace and harmony in the kingdom." While the kidney provides the power for the whole organ system to function, the heart provides its soul. Every organ needs Qi to function, and it also needs the right message or organizing force.

This message comes from the heart. Your heart's job is to animate all the organs, maintain their proper function, and enable them to come together and act in concert, like one exquisite symphony. Your heart, as well as your liver, performs an aspect of controlling the circulation of blood, but also has another assignment: it controls aspects of your mind and emotions.

In the Five Element Theory, the heart's partner organ is the small intestine. Its element is fire. The opening gate to the outside of the body is the tongue. The tissue it controls are the blood vessels. The emotion that can affect the heart is joy. The seasonal energy and time which matches the heart's is summer. Its environmental factor is heat. The color related to heart energy is red. The taste that goes directly to the heart is bitter. The direction or location is South.

The Heart and the Kidney

More than any other organ, the heart must have strong kidney support (if you go back and look at the Five Element Theory Chart, you will see that the kidney controls the heart). Palpitations in menopause, for example, are usually a signal that your heart's function is out of balance with your kidney. It's not that you don't have a sufficient blood supply, rather, TCM says that there isn't enough Qi or power to help keep the heart functioning as it should. Consequently, your heart must pump more forcefully to keep your blood moving. Strong Qi is essential to good circulation.

As you may know, in the West, heart disease is the leading cause of death among post-menopausal women. Why? From the

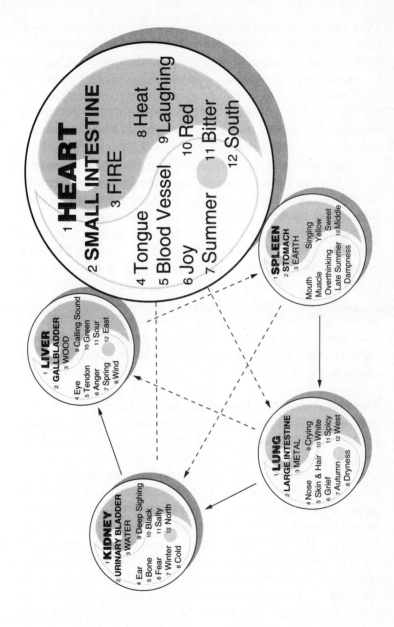

TCM standpoint, menopausal women who develop heart disease have a kidney Qi deficiency. From what you now know about In-born Qi, you undoubtedly recognize that older people in general are more susceptible to heart problems because their kidney Qi has naturally declined with age. During our later years, the kidney has less Qi to draw on to do its proper job of cooling the heart or controlling its fire. Basically, your heart will overheat if your kidney is too weak to cool it down.

Your heart also controls body fluids. TCM says "perspiration is the liquid of the heart." If you perspire too much and too often, your heart may have a Qi deficiency problem, or conversely, this excessive loss of fluid can cause a Qi deficiency of the heart. This is why you may want to rethink your exercise routine, especially if it makes you perspire too much. By trying to improve your cardiovascular health, you may actually be impairing it. According to TCM, sweating too much is definitely not a good thing; neither is excessive exercising. Once in a while, we are shocked by the death of a younger athlete who succumbs to a sudden heart attack. If exercise is supposed to help protect the heart, then why do these seemingly healthy people leave us too soon?

The Heart and the Pericardium

Because too much heat can be such a problem for the heart, it has a special guardian in the pericardium. Physically, the pericardium is the membranous sac that surrounds the heart. Its job is to "defend" your heart and help prevent it from overheating. Some signs of an overheated heart are a dry mouth, thirst (especially at night), cold sores, and yellow urine. Skin breakouts and night-mares are also signs of this condition. Heart fire has the ability to affect your digestion because the heart and small intestine are an organ pair that communicate through Qi and share a close energy connection. Therefore, an overheated heart can pass its fire along to the small intestine, whose own job is to play an important role in absorbing nutrition from food. Too much heat in the small in-testine then creates a Qi imbalance that can then cause poor digestion, make your body feel uncomfortably full, or produce that infamous symptom—heartburn!

The Heart and the Liver

The heart also shares another close energy relationship with the liver, its "mother." When your liver is overstressed, its Qi is pulled elsewhere and cannot support your heart's work. Your liver not only supplies your heart with blood, it plays an important role in circulation, ensuring that the flow of blood is smooth and steady. In TCM theory, the three major organs having to do with blood are the heart, liver, and spleen: the heart governs all activities of the blood, the liver stores blood and regulates its flow, and the spleen creates both Qi and blood from the essence of food, and controls the blood as well. This intricate web of connections keeps blood moving properly throughout your body and it helps your heart, and consequently your whole body, function smoothly.

Cause of Heart Problems

Heart problems are the number one cause of death for women in the United States after the age of fifty. According to the American Heart Association, more than 250,000 women die each year from heart-related problems. In all, about three times as many women die from heart disease as they do from breast cancer. The cause of some heart problems can be difficult to pinpoint. High blood pressure, for example, can be related to the heart, the kidney, or the stomach. As always in TCM, it is essential to identify which organ (or combination of organs) is the real troublemaker. But in the case of high blood pressure, the root cause is generally a combination of organs. High blood pressure is not a simple problem, because it develops when there is a functional disorder of all the organs. In the case of high blood pressure, the entire body is out of balance. I've talked about the two types of Qi or energies in the body, yin and yang. The flow of each must follow its natural direction: yang Qi goes up and yin Qi goes down. TCM didn't make this up; it is the natural law governing the movement of Qi. In an individual with high blood pressure, this doesn't happen. Too much Qi rises, where it gets stuck in the head. To treat high blood pressure, TCM will treat this upset in the imbalance of the body's energy system, and try to get the whole body back in harmony.

High cholesterol and clogged arteries are other examples of function problems whose origins can reside in multiple organs. Most often, their root cause is in your liver. When any or all of the organs function poorly, your body gradually loses its self-regulating capabilities and falls out of balance. (When your body is well, it manages cholesterol levels very nicely and keeps your arteries open.) This is true even if the organs themselves are fine physically. The body then becomes inefficient and sluggish. Substances such as fat, water, and toxins tend to accumulate. It is vital, at this point, to identify why your body is falling out of harmony. In other words, TCM will still search for the root cause, rather than just treat its symptoms.

Complex problems like high blood pressure or high cholesterol do not receive disease-specific treatment from TCM. In fact, TCM does not even categorize these problems in Western medical terms. As you've learned by now, a skilled TCM doctor will analyze a patient's individual symptoms; then, diagnosis and treatment will focus on the organs determined to be the root cause. In contrast, Western medicine might approach these conditions by trying to suppress or control their symptoms with medication. It will tend to isolate or divide the problem into parts and treat the parts. For instance, the side effects from taking high blood pressure medication may be offset with additional drugs. These drugs, in turn, can cause their own side effects, and so on. TCM does not separate a patient from his or her symptoms, it views the person as an integrated whole. It always looks at the larger picture of the condition of the body's energy system, as well as the body's relationship with the Universe. Over millennia, TCM has utilized a vast body of experience and knowledge to bring a body back into harmony. When this is accomplished, a person can heal herself.

The Heart as Keeper of the Spirit

As king of all organs, the heart houses the *Shen* or spirit. It also houses the control center for the other four aspects of the soul, which reside in the lung, spleen, liver, and kidney. TCM considers your heart to be the ruler of all mental activities. When TCM speaks of the mind, it has a broader meaning than that in the West. It includes aspects of consciousness in the concept of "mental activities" that include intelligence and thinking; memory and sleep; emotions, as well as the various aspects of the soul.

In TCM's view, most mental and sleep problems can be traced straight to the source—unbalanced heart Qi. Because the heart relates specifically to intelligence, TCM recognizes that meditation can be applied to help relieve emotional distress. However, if your heart is weak or overheated as described earlier, or if it is not supplied with enough blood, your spirit cannot rest peacefully there. If you're going through menopause, I think you will recognize many of the health conditions that my patients experience. They describe their whole body as feeling uneasy and restless. They say that their thinking becomes cloudy or fuzzy, and their memory is poor. (Naturally, this causes them to become stressful, as they begin to worry about having early Alzheimer's disease.) Insomnia and nightmares may occur.

Have you ever had a night when your mind seems to float, or worse, to race? Many of my patients talk about their mind "racing" at night when they are trying desperately to get to sleep. Do you ever feel like you are asleep, yet you're aware of being awake at the same time? For ages, TCM has viewed these conditions as an indication that your heart is unable to "house" your *Shen* or spirit. If you want to feel calm, think clearly, and sleep soundly, you must take care of your heart. Above all, if you can keep your heart in a joyful, peaceful state, you can also help reduce the effect of stress on the all-important liver. Why? Because this way the "child" can please its "mother."

Taking Care of Your Heart

What can you do to take care of your heart? First, it is helpful to understand that the organ itself has powers and ability far beyond its physical structure. Think about how powerful your heart is because it relates to unconditional love. Real love comes from your heart, not your mind. One of the very important purposes of the *Wu Ming* Meridian Therapy in Chapter 13 is to help you open your heart. TCM believes this kind of physical and spiritual energy practice definitely can help keep your heart well. In Eastern philosophy, many texts talk about meditation and emptying the mind. When the mind is empty, the heart can finally rest. It can conserve its own spirit or *Shen,* as well as its physical Qi. If your mind is always in motion, you should remember that your spirit is in motion as well. It is when your mind is empty that your heart can truly open. If you can reach this state, then unconditional love and forgiveness can enter. You can forget the past and move on. Enormous burdens that we carry can dissolve this way. TCM believes that when a heart offers unconditional love, it can reach infinity. We all know that love is the best way to nurture and heal the heart. Smiling and being happy may sound too simple and too easy, but this time-tested wisdom brings us a real truth. Menopause presents an ideal time to strengthen and protect your heart. Remember this transition is your final opportunity to get truly healthy for the wonderful journey ahead. Take the time to practice opening your heart. When you slow down and quiet your mind, you can forget about the self. When you forget about the self, you have the opportunity to heal your heart and touch the part of you that is eternal. I urge you to practice *Wu Ming* Meridian Therapy as often as you can. The benefits are tremendous.

The Western way to strengthen the heart involves cardiovascular exercises; the Eastern way is to harbor peaceful thoughts and keep the mind empty. Meditation makes your heart worry less and become more peaceful. The TCM way to keep your heart healthy involves: working at keeping all your organs functioning in harmony; trying not to overuse your mental faculties; maintaining a positive, happy, and accepting outlook at all times.

Here is one of the most powerful ancient exercises you can do for your heart. Face the mirror and smile at yourself—really smile at yourself—from your heart. How simple this may seem, yet how difficult this practice is for most people. Smiling from your heart—not just a fake smile—actually has a physical effect. It can help make blood and Qi flow throughout your whole body. When you've mastered this practice, then try smiling at others from your heart. We know that smiling and laughter can create emotional Qi and propel it through the body to help it heal. This practice helps heal the heart. From my experience, I believe it's much more effective than physical exercise.

It's interesting to see how many phrases relating to the true power of the heart are used unconsciously in Western society . I'm sure you're familiar with many of them. We say: "You broke my heart." We don't say: "You broke my mind." Is your physical heart really broken? No, but if you've ever really had your heart broken, you know something deep within you beyond the physical has been deeply wounded or affected. When we say: "You're in my heart," does this mean that your whole body is in someone else's heart? No. It means that you carry their spirit with you. Even the popular song from the movie *Titanic,* is titled "My Heart Will Go On," not "My Mind Will Go On." It reflects the concept held by so many spiritual and philosophical practices that the heart's spirit lives on with its memories and experiences, even though the body may perish.

Here's some interesting observations about the aging process that relate to the heart and the kidney. Though older people may not remember yesterday or today's activities, they can remember things that happened in the distant past very clearly. This is related to the heart's activity of memory. Many older people have difficulty sleeping in their own beds, but you can find them falling asleep continually in their own comfortable chair in front of the television. This is related to the heart's activity of sleep. If you speak very loudly to some older people, you will find that they have difficulty hearing you, but if you carry on a phone conversation, interestingly, they can overhear whatever you say. This is related to the heart's activity of intelligence. Also, you may find that older people have less sexual desire; however, they have more desire for being loved. If they are not loved or do not feel loved, jealousy is often the outcome.

Finally, we've seen that smiling is related to the heart. You may have seen for yourself that when older people are sad, they cry, but no tears come. That's because sadness is the lung's emotion and its partnership with the kidney has weakened with the aging process, so producing tears is difficult. When older people are happy and smiling, often they can't control the flow of tears. That's because tears are the "liquid of the heart" and happiness or joy is its emotion. Again, a weakened kidney cannot control the flow. These are age-related examples of unbalanced relationships: first between the kidney and lung, then between the kidney and the heart.

THE SPLEEN, THE GENERATOR OF QI

One of TCM's most ancient Chinese physicians put forth the theory that "all human health problems are initially caused by a spleen/stomach dysfunction."

In the Five Element Theory, the spleen's element is earth. The opening gate to the outside of the body is the mouth. The tissue it controls is the muscle. The emotions that can affect the spleen are overthinking and anxiety. The spleen's partner organ is the stomach. The seasonal energy and time which matches the spleen is late summer. Its environmental factor is dampness. The color related to spleen energy is yellow. The taste that goes directly to the spleen is sweet. The direction or location is Middle.

Proper functioning of the digestive system depends on the spleen, which—with its partner the stomach, is the body's main source of Qi after birth. This is the most important way our bodies receive "income" to deposit in our energy or checking account of Acquired Qi. Remember, it is from this account that your body's daily Qi expenditures should be drawn. This is where the body gets the Qi it needs to digest food and liquid. Your stomach re-

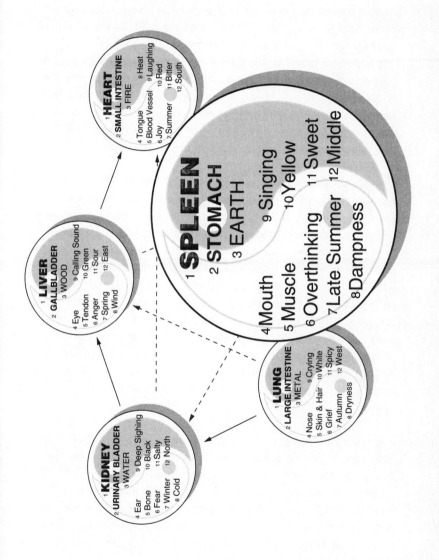

ceives these things and "rots and ripens" them, as TCM theory puts it. Your spleen then transforms this mixture into a refined essence called "*gu* Qi." This food essence forms the material foundation of your Qi and blood. Thus, the daily fuel and nourishment for your whole body depends on the spleen and stomach enjoying a healthy cooperative partnership. This is a lifetime linkage that must be kept strong. If the organs themselves function weakly, or if their partnership isn't strong, or if eating habits become poor—or both, as is often the case—the body will not be properly nourished. Then you can suffer from both deficient Qi and deficient blood.

Problems from Deficient Spleen/Stomach Qi

Because deficient Qi has the ability to destabilize the function of your other organs, TCM puts a lot of emphasis on keeping your spleen and stomach in good shape. Deficient blood not only affects your liver, but also your heart. As we have seen, it can cause problems like palpitations and insomnia. Anemia, dry skin and hair, and fatigue are other signs that your spleen cannot produce sufficient blood. Other signals I recommend you pay attention to are poor muscle tone or weak, aching muscles. In TCM theory, your spleen governs the muscles, which depend upon strong spleen Qi and blood for nourishment. Your hands and feet are under the control of the spleen. If the spleen has a problem, you might notice that your extremities are always cold, or they sweat constantly. Cellulite is also a spleen problem.

The natural flow of spleen Qi is upward: it sends food essence up to the lung for distribution and holds your body's organs and tissues in place. A weak spleen cannot perform these functions very well. Spleen problems tend to be ones of deficiency—the spleen seldom suffers from problems of excess. When your spleen Qi is so weak that it sinks instead of rises, certain organs can sink as well, especially the stomach, intestines, uterus, and rectum. Other symptoms of weak, sinking Qi are diarrhea, fatigue, and blurred vision.

Your spleen has another important job. Besides transporting food essence, it also ferries fluids throughout the body. A Qi-deficient or weak spleen does not have the power to properly regulate all the fluids in your body. This is not good because weak spleen function can lead to excessive dampness. This is the organ that especially dislikes any kind of dampness because this environmental factor interferes with its work of transforming and transporting your nutritive essence. Poor spleen function can cause a range of digestive problems: lack of appetite, poor digestion, loose stool or diarrhea, and abdominal distention. It can also cause you to retain water and gain weight.

Weight is a major issue for people in the West. The statistics on obesity, even for children, are alarming. Consumers are spending billions of dollars on programs and products of all kinds to lose weight. If you have trouble losing weight, the problem may be your spleen. Look at your tongue. If it is fat, with a thick white coating, it is a signal that your body is unable to rid itself of excess water. I tell my patients to be careful about trying to lose weight. Dieting can further weaken spleen Qi and make the problem of ridding your body of excess water more difficult.

Even if you lose weight, if your spleen does not have enough Qi, you're apt not only to gain it back, but you will have more trouble losing it again. TCM says that overeating is not the cause of this kind of weight problem; it is a function disorder. In the Dragon's Way®, my Center's self-healing weight loss program, I concentrate first on improving the functions of the spleen and stomach and then helping this all-important partnership come back into harmony. When this happens, the body loses weight naturally.

Today, I have close to one thousand Dragon's Way® graduates who can attest to the effectiveness of this healthy and healing approach to weight loss. The complete Dragon's Way program is outlined in another book in our series on TCM. It is called *Traditional Chinese Medicine: A Natural Guide to Weight Loss That Lasts* (HarperCollins 2000). In our program, the goal is to increase the body's Qi. Remember that most diets decrease, not increase, your body's Qi. Also, if you are serious about losing weight, you must learn how to eat for healing—to avoid cold foods such as salads and raw vegetables, for example. For women of menopausal age, there are some key foods that are very beneficial for this period in your life. I strongly urge you to study Chapter 15. Think about this: if you have reached the age of menopause, your kidney Qi or energy foundation is already declining, according to the natural law. If you don't get enough quality Qi for your life's daily activities from the foods you eat, where will this extra Qi come from? By now, you know it will come directly from your kidney Qi. The bigger the deficit of Acquired Qi in your energy checking account; the bigger the raid on your irreplaceable energy savings account of Inborn Qi. The result? The steeper and faster the aging process occurs; the more symptoms emerge; the faster the ultimate destination is reached. That's really the way it works. Have you ever noticed how different women look from one another when they enter the menopause years? Some remain vibrant and healthy looking; some appear to be a decade older than they really are. You can really begin to tell which women have taken care of themselves at this time. Luckily, for the others there is still an opportunity to help themselves.

The spleen controls the flow of blood, how it flows, where it flows and how much blood should flow into a given body structure. The liver too relates to blood circulation, but its interest is only in storing blood and making sure it flows freely. It has no interest in controlling blood flow. It just delivers the blood.

If the spleen has a problem, there will usually be conditions of internal bleeding. Women with poor spleen function may experience an abnormally long menstrual cycle or spotting between periods. A lot of menopausal women also suffer from frequent spotting and excessive bleeding. Hysterectomies are often performed as a solution to this problem. In my opinion, this is a procedure that is frequently unnecessary. According to TCM, the true root cause of excessive bleeding is not the uterus or ovaries, but deficient spleen Qi.

The tone and elasticity of blood vessel walls is also the spleen's job. If the organ is too weak to perform this function, your blood vessel walls can become fragile and even collapse. This may cause bruising, varicose veins, and chronic bleeding. Fixing this problem means going to the source and helping the spleen regain its ability to function normally.

Often, menopausal patients who are bleeding excessively need only a few TCM treatments to achieve very good results. In my practice, I use special herbal formulas adapted specifically for my Western patients and acupuncture to help women stop this kind of bleeding and save their uterus in the process. Naturally, this is very important to my younger patients in their childbearing years. If they continue to take good care of themselves in their twenties and thirties, they can help themselves avoid future problems as they encounter perimenopause and when they go through the menopause years.

While your heart houses the *Shen*, your spleen offers a home to the *Yi*—the aspect of the soul that provides the capacity for applied thinking, concentration, and some functions of memory. Too much thinking or worrying excessively (the spleen's corresponding emotion) can actually deplete your spleen's Qi. They can also lead to depression, one of our society's major problems. In Western culture, depression is frequently treated with drugs like the popular Prozac or Zoloft and many others. Often these antidepressants can cause side effects that affect the stomach.

A lot of my women patients ask me if TCM has a way to help alleviate depression without drug therapy. Many of them are eager to discontinue these drugs. My response is that to address this condition, they must fix the underlying imbalance in the spleen's function first. I advise them to consult their doctors before stopping any medication. (I also always advise my patients to let their doctors know that they are taking herbal formulas.) Then, together we work out a plan to treat the spleen by changing their diet and adding foods that help heal the spleen; identifying lifestyle habits that must be improved, and using acupuncture to help the liver function more smoothly. There is also one classical Chinese formula in use for centuries that I have adapted for my Western patients. This combination of natural treatments has proved very effective in helping my patients deal with the root cause of their depression.

For many women, excessive thinking and worry are also coupled with poor eating habits. When these conditions occur, a double blow is delivered to a smoothly operating spleen/stomach partnership. Long before a woman reaches menopause, her spleen may have been weakened substantially by these critical factors, resulting in many of the symptoms outlined above. TCM does everything possible to save the spleen if it has a problem; it does not view this as a disposable organ. TCM believes that the spleen plays an essential role in an individual's overall well-being and longevity.

THE IMPORTANCE OF THE STOMACH

Before we move on to the lung, I want to help you understand the spleen's companion organ, the stomach, from the TCM perspective. TCM considers your stomach a bowel, that is, it fills up with food and water, digests and transforms these materials, then empties itself. These activities don't occur by themselves. They are powered by your stomach's Qi, on which TCM places tremendous importance. While the kidney powers the internal functions of each individual organ, it is sufficient stomach Qi that gives each of the organs enough power to perform its job. A deficiency of stomach Qi can lead to weakness in all of the organs. As we've seen, a properly functioning stomach working in cooperation with your spleen supports the daily activities of your body. According to TCM theory, whether or not your body can recover from illness or disease also depends on a strong spleen/stomach partnership.

From my experience, stomach problems—either of deficiency or excess—are always connected to liver function problems. These two organs share a control relationship and the liver will strive to keep their relationship in balance. If the stomach suffers from a Qi deficiency, then naturally, digestive problems will follow. Here are a few signs that will help you identify a stomach Qi deficiency:

- You feel relief from your stomach pains after you eat;
- You experience stomach bloating and loose stool;

- You have a fat tongue with a white coating;
- Your hands and feet always feel cold;
- You bruise easily;
- You are overweight.

Generally speaking, if your stomach pain goes away if you rest, massage it, or eat something warm, your condition is one of deficiency. In the case of a Qi deficiency, make sure you avoid cold food and cold fluids, as much as possible. Stomach Qi deficiency can also cause hypoglycemia and migraine headaches. In this case, the migraine headache will usually occur across the front of the forehead, which is where the stomach meridian runs. Here are some foods that bring warmth to the stomach and spleen:

ANCIENT TCM TIP FOR SELF-HEALING

Foods That Bring Warmth to the Stomach and Spleen.

1. Cinnamon
2. Ginger
3. Fennel seeds
4. Garlic
5. Black and white pepper
6. Chinese barley (from a Chinese food store)

According to natural law, your stomach loves warmth. Its function can become unbalanced or suffer from Qi deficiency if you continually feed it a diet of cold food, uncooked food (like raw vegetables or salads), or cold fluids (like ice water and soda). So be kind to your stomach and keep it warm!

Some individuals, on the other hand, have stomachs that suffer from a condition of excess heat caused by liver Qi that stagnates in the stomach. They experience a different set of problems such as burping, rib and stomach distention, and stomach pain. Often they have a sour taste in their mouth (associated with the liver), or persistent bad breath. Their tongue will have a yellow coating. They may even be continually constipated. If these conditions occur, it is important to treat the liver as well as the stomach, otherwise the root cause remains. Often this excess heat comes from an internal source such as emotional problems like continually held anger and relentless stress. Excess heat can also result from external sources like eating too much fried or spicy foods, and drinking too much alcohol. This condition also has the ability to cause a migraine headache in the forehead as well as TMJ. Gums that bleed or swell are also related to excess stomach heat.

THE LUNG: BREATHING THE BREATH OF LIFE

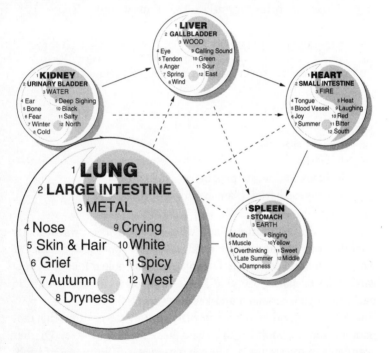

One of your lung's primary functions is the control of your whole body's Qi. In the Five Element Theory, the lung's partner organ is the large intestine. Its element is metal. The opening gate to the outside of the body is the nose. The tissues it controls are the skin and body hair. The emotion that can affect the lung is grief or sadness. The seasonal energy and time which matches the lung's is autumn. Its environmental factor is dryness. The color related to lung energy is white. The taste that goes directly to the lung is pungent or spicy. The direction or location is West.

From its high position in the chest, your lung governs both the formation of Qi, which occurs within the lung, as well as the distribution of Qi throughout the body. Inhaled air combines with food essence sent to your lung from the spleen, its "mother," or energy generating organ. The resulting *zong* Qi, which is a kind of a master Qi, then becomes the basis for other types of Qi, which are sent like messengers traveling throughout your body to nourish, moisten, warm, and protect it. All of this happens, of course, in less than the blink of an eye during the "automatic transfer" process of the healthy body we discussed in the Theory of Yin and Yang.

Wei Qi (or defensive Qi as it is known), for instance, is dispersed by the lung to the area between the muscles and skin to warm and guard the body's surface. TCM believes that external pathogens such as wind, cold, and heat invade your body through the skin. Your skin is your first line of defense and it is your lung's job to keep this protective mechanism working well. Weak lung Qi impairs this protective function and leaves your body vulnerable to a variety of problems, including increased susceptibility to colds and flu. This may be particularly apparent to you if you always get sick in the fall, the season that the lung rules.

One way to conserve lung Qi is to dress warmly as the weather becomes cooler in the autumn. Windy days should be regarded as an enemy of good health since wind is the external pathogen with the most power to break through the body's first line of defense—the skin's energy barrier. Because other pathogens often attach themselves to wind, they too, can invade your body. No matter what season, TCM views wind as a serious external problem to be vigilantly guarded against. For instance, you might think nothing of shedding your sweater on a warm fall day. I advise my patients not to do this because the nature of fall's energy is always cool. Simply putting on a sweater or jacket goes a long way toward saving your lung from spending extra *wei* Qi to warm and protect your body. It is important during menopause to save as much Qi as possible. If you have or have had breast cancer, you also must accumulate as much *wei* Qi as possible to spend on self-healing. This is an example of finding everyday opportunities where you have control over building up your healing Qi.

In addition to invading your body through the skin, external pathogens can also enter through your mouth and nose (the "opening" of the lung). Your lung is the only internal organ in direct contact with the exterior world, which makes it extremely vulnerable to external pathogens. TCM refers to the lung as a "baby organ" because it is so delicate. When your lung is invaded by cold, for instance, you may suffer from cold symptoms such as congestion, sneezing, and coughing. The TCM approach to treating a cough caused by external cold is to try to push it out of the body. This contrasts with the Western approach which tries to "kill" or suppress the cough with a variety of pills, syrups, and nasal decongestants.

Here's an interesting example of what can actually happen when a cough gets suppressed.

I have one patient who is a graphic designer in his late thirties. He came to me to try and cure a terrible skin problem on his hands and arms. The condition, which looked very bad, made everyone afraid to shake hands with him. If he handed over money, people were reluctant to take it. The fluid released by scratching his hands would often cause his girlfriend to have an allergic reaction. By the time I saw him, he was desperate and willing to try almost anything because he had had this condition for more than ten years. He had been to many dermatologists and taken many internal and external remedies. Nothing helped.

At first, I used certain TCM treatments to treat this problem as a typical skin condition. Although this helped somewhat, his skin condition continued to come and go. Then, I asked him if he could recall what happened in his life before this skin condition appeared. He related that he remembered having a severe cough for a few months for which antibiotics were prescribed. When his cough stopped, his hand started to develop a kind of eczema. He could actually remember the site where his skin problem first developed, which I recognized immediately as an area on the lung meridian. Using TCM theory, I diagnosed this situation as one where the cough's energy was trying to break out of the body through its skin.

I told him that I was going to change his herbal formula and that he might experience a cough. I told him not to worry about this cough because we would be allowing this old problem a way out of his body. Shortly he began to experience the cough we expected. In just a few weeks though, his long-time skin problem began to show remarkable improvement. We continued this treatment for a few months. His hands and arms healed completely. This was about five years ago, and the problem has never returned. This case is an ideal example of how TCM theory can pinpoint the root cause of a difficult health problem. Without understanding the principles and theories of this ancient medicine, I must admit the treatment direction might seem a little strange.

The Lung as Manager of Qi and Nutrition

TCM also sees the lung as the "manager" of Qi and nutrition. We've seen how your spleen performs its job of sending the essence or energy of food upward to the lung. We've also described above how the lung, in turn, parcels this Qi out to the other organs. Good digestion is vital to this process, so is eating good quality food. Your lung also plays a part in promoting the circulation of blood. While your heart controls your blood vessels, your lung helps create the energy to push blood through them. If your lung is weak, circulation will be poor, and your body will not be properly warmed and nourished. Symptoms of insufficient lung Qi include cough and shortness of breath, cold limbs and hands, sweating, and fatigue. Your lung is also a key player when it comes to the body's metabolism of water. It directs your body's water downward to the kidney and urinary bladder for elimination. Weak lung function can cause urinary problems or water retention (if you tend to be overweight, you may be suffering from lung Qi deficiency). And because your lung has a close energy relationship with its partner, the large intestine, constipation and diarrhea can also have their origins in poor lung function.

The Lung and Luminous Skin

TCM says that part of your lung's job as the manager of nutrition is to send fluids to your skin to nourish and moisten it. According to the Five Element Theory, your skin is the body tissue governed by your lung; the condition of the skin reflects the strength and quality of this organ's Qi. Deficient lung Qi can manifest itself in dry, rough, itchy skin.

What about wrinkles and other signs of aging that show up in the skin, especially in the face? One of the benefits of taking estrogen is said to be that it reduces signs of aging, especially wrinkles, crow's feet, etc. TCM, however, sees skin condition relating not just to your age, but to the quality of lung Qi specifically, and the overall level of Qi generally. TCM believes that wherever there are wrinkles, there is an insufficient amount of nourishment and Qi to support muscle and skin health. Furthermore, with the six major Yang meridians running through the face, having a face-lift cuts through these vital meridians and can damage them severely. It's like cutting off the roots of a tree. You may look better initially, but it's almost inevitable that some unwanted problems will develop later. This is why TCM's holistic approach concentrates primarily on reducing the signs of aging from the inside out. External treatment may offer some benefit, but there is nothing as powerful (or as attractive!) as letting good health shine from within.

The lung is also home to the *Po,* the physical aspect of its soul. TCM believes this soul stays in the earth after death. The *Po* controls all the physical and mental activities of your five senses. This includes smelling, hearing, tasting, and touch and all movement, whether of your limbs or your thoughts. If you have trouble with your balance, most likely your lung is not functioning properly. Your lung is like the assistant who carries out the orders of the chief executive; anything that requires movement depends upon your lung Qi functioning smoothly. Your lung is also the first organ to die. Because the lung controls all of the Qi, or life force, that you have built up after birth, when this critical organ expires, so do you.

Remember that we said that each of the twelve meridians is "on duty" for two hours at a time in the body. The lung is the first organ "in charge." Its hours are from 3:00 A.M. to 5:00 A.M. It is not surprising then that most hospital deaths are recorded during this time period. Individuals who are critically ill simply do not have enough lung Qi to go on. If they can weather this crucial time period, however, it means that their body has enough Qi or energy to fight another day to try and heal itself.

ANCIENT TCM TIP FOR SELF-HEALING

Six Foods You Can Add to Your Diet to Increase Lung Qi.

1. Almonds
2. Pears
3. Persimmons
4. Honey
5. Lily bulb (from a Chinese food store)
6. White mushrooms (not the American kind, but from a Chinese food store)

THE KIDNEY: YOUR ENERGY FOUNDATION

I've saved the kidney for last because by this time you should be very familiar with this organ and its role as the body's power engine. Because we've talked about the kidney all through this chapter, I'll spend a short time filling in some things you don't already know.

In the Five Element Theory, the kidney's partner organ is the bladder. Its element is water. The opening gate to the outside of the body is the ear. The tissue it controls is the bone. The emotions that can affect the kidney are fear and shock. The seasonal energy and time that matches the kidney's is winter. Its environ-

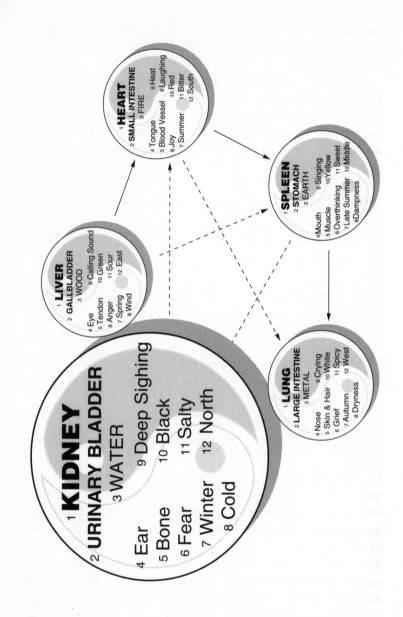

mental factor is cold. The color related to kidney energy is black. The taste that goes directly to the kidney is salty. The direction or location is North.

On the cosmic ladder to the Tao, the kidney's *Jing* Qi plays a significant role. In TCM practice, there are three major elements that directly influence human life: *Jing* or "life-essence"; Qi or life force; *Shen* or life spirit. The *Nei Jing* says that if you can maintain the *Shen*, then you can have life; if you lose your *Shen* or life spirit, then it is time to die.

TCM also uses this concept to explain one of its deeper principles—attaining ultimate spiritual harmony between the human and the Universe. It even sets down the path for us: accumulate *Jing* first, then transmute *Jing* to Qi. Accumulate Qi and then transmute it into *Shen*. Accumulate *Shen* and transmute it into emptiness. Then transmute emptiness to the Tao where you can become one with the Universe. The *Wu Ming* Meridian Therapy Qigong movements in this book offer one of the most effective paths for reaching this goal. Again, I urge you to consider how lucky you are to reach this transitional time in your life and to realize how deepening your spiritual side can have an amazing affect on your health and healing.

As we've said, the kidney's main job is to generate power for the entire body. Its other job is to store the *Jing* or concentrated life-essence. It is within the *Jing* Qi that the two essential components of Inborn Qi and Acquired Qi reside. As you've already seen, we are constantly drawing on our savings account of Inborn Qi, and often use its precious funds wastefully. So remember, you must do everything you can to conserve it. Conservation, if we follow the way of nature, is the most important principle with regard to the kidney. The kidney, of course, corresponds with the season of winter. And think of what happens during the winter. Nature withdraws into herself, she saves her energy, she rests. In the same way, especially if you are going through menopause, you must recognize the value of your energy foundation and do everything possible to conserve it.

The *Nei Jing* says, "The sage knows that *Jing*/Essence is the most precious substance in the body. Like the root of a tree, it should be protected and hidden from thieves." What are these energy thieves? For certain, stress and overwork are two of them. Also, one of the biggest thieves of kidney Qi is sex. It's important to note that sexual activity draws heavily on kidney Qi. Sex, in moderation, is a good and healthy activity at any age. But, it makes the heart beat faster, and the whole body function at a very high rate of Qi expenditure. (And, the Qi that it is drawing on just happens to be your irreplaceable Inborn Qi.) If your energy foundation is not strong, it isn't advisable, nor is it smart, to weaken it further with excessive sexual activity.

Ways to Slow the Kidney's Energy Decline

While it may not be easy to increase kidney Qi, slowing its decline is another matter, and there are many ways you can do this. Conserving Qi is the number one way. Practicing the ancient self-healing art of Qigong is another, because it can help the body rebalance itself and bring it up to its maximum functioning capability. Following a good diet with high-quality foods is another important step. Below are foods you can eat that help boost the power of the kidney. It's especially important to make these foods a part of your diet during the winter months when the kidney is most susceptible to problems. When I lecture, I tell my audiences that Qi is like money in some ways. One way to increase wealth is to go out and add new sums. Another way is to cut expenses. As we've seen, TCM considers it almost impossible to acquire more Inborn Qi, but it is possible to cut our Qi expenditures and conserve Qi for longevity. For menopausal women, I highly recommend eating these foods.

ANCIENT TCM TIP FOR SELF-HEALING

Five foods you can eat to help boost kidney Qi.

1. Shellfish: lobster, shrimp, clams, oysters; seafood of all kinds

2. Beans: especially black ones
3. Bone marrow and bone marrow soup
4. Walnuts (roasted)
5. Pine nuts

Strengthening your kidney also helps prevent the loss of Qi through poor organ function or using your Qi up to repair "broken" connections among the organs. This reduces the amount of Qi your body must use to function well. Of particular importance, of course, is balancing the body to ensure that the spleen and stomach are able to produce more Qi from food. This is like cost avoidance; it enables you to reduce the amount of Qi that you need to draw from your kidney. Here's how this works. Let's say that you need one hundred units of Qi every day for your body to function. This Qi ideally should come from the spleen and stomach. However, if they cannot produce the required amount, the kidney has to make up the balance. So poor digestive function is another energy thief, stealing the kidney's limited treasure.

The Kidney and Brain Power

You know by now that the root cause behind many menopausal and postmenopausal problems is poor kidney function. I've already talked about the importance of the kidney in taking care of the heart, and in maintaining strong healthy bones. There's another area where TCM understands the kidney's essential role: brain function.

You may have heard the latest argument for the use of estrogen is that it may help reduce the risk of or delay the onset of Alzheimer's disease. TCM, however, looks at it this way. It states that both the heart and kidney control mental activity. The heart, as king of the organs, exerts a direct control, while the kidney's influence is indirect. The kidney governs the bones and the marrow. The brain, in TCM, is called the "sea of marrow," because bone marrow—especially of the spine—supports the brain and all of its functions. Therefore, TCM believes that good memory function is related to strong kidney Qi. As kidney Qi declines with age, the power of memory tends to diminish as well. In extreme cases, such as Alzheimer's, the function of the brain breaks down altogether.

Other Signs of Weak Kidney Qi

There are many other signs that tell you your kidney Qi is weakening. You may feel cold all the time, a cold that comes from the inside. You may lose your hair or your sex drive, common problems that arrive with age. The ears are the "opening" of the kidney, and are sustained by its Qi, so if your kidney Qi weakens, your ears may start to ring, or you may suffer from earaches or lose your hearing.

Your bones are under the control of the kidney. Bones will definitely become brittle and weaken as kidney Qi declines. If you have weak or sore knees, if you have heel pain, if you suffer from bone spurs, these are all signs of weak kidney Qi. TCM calls the teeth "the surplus of the bone." If you have problems with your teeth, or they start to fall out, your body is exhibiting signs of weakened kidney Qi.

Another common symptom related to deficient kidney Qi is lower back pain that is not due to an injury. Estimates are that 50 to 80 percent of Americans complain of back problems during their lifetimes. Why? TCM understands that the lower back is the house of the kidney. If the foundation is shaky, how can the house be strong? A woman might experience some of these symptoms well before menopause, because in a stress-filled culture her kidney Qi often begins to drop around age thirty-five. My hope is that by understanding the significance of these signs you will begin to take better care of yourself starting right now. I also hope that the younger you are the more you'll do to prevent problems today so you can live a long, healthy life tomorrow.

As a woman, you are lucky in a very special way. In addition to your kidney, you have a second "engine" that generates Qi or vital energy: this is your uterus and ovaries. These extra organs are unique because they are able to receive, store, and accumulate Qi. Just as a baby is conceived, matures in the womb, and is then delivered, the Qi in this "engine" grows and then empties itself. This Qi transfer happens monthly during your menstrual cycle. Within this natural rhythm, you accumulate Qi, Qi becomes blood, and the blood then passes from your body. Thus you have an innate or in-born natural skill that helps you tune up your body every single month of your menstruating years. Your uterus and ovaries are also the engine that produces hormones throughout your child-bearing years. And TCM believes that even after menopause, if you are healthy, your reproductive organs can still function as a Qi engine, and continue to produce the hormones you need. After menopause, these special organs do need more support, however, and must produce hormones in cooperation with your kidney.

I'd like to stress once again the importance of not removing the uterus (hysterectomy) or ovaries (oophorectomy), if at all possible. Data show that women who have had a hysterectomy have more problems going through menopause. Be very careful about having your unique gift taken from you. If you suffer from problems such as excessive bleeding, and the cause is a Qi deficiency—not tumors or cancer—classical Chinese herbal formulas can help you. In my experience, just three to five days of this kind of herbal therapy can be enough to stop the bleeding. Even after menopause, your reproductive organs retain their power or Qi; they still carry their own message of hormone production. And, most importantly, they can still play their part in the integrated system that creates overall Qi to support your body's health.

Now that you have a solid foundation on TCM, we're ready to talk specifics about how you can reestablish yourself as "mistress" of your own manor.

TO SUMMARIZE:

- When TCM talks about an organ, it is referring not only to a physical structure but to a whole complex of functions that are both physiological and psychological. It refers to the lung and the kidney in the singular to emphasize this larger meaning.
- According to the Five Element Theory, each organ

governs a body tissue and a sense organ, is related to a particular emotion, houses one of the five aspects of the soul, and has a partner organ.

- All the organs have a Qi connection with each other through the Meridian network.
- As long as you can keep your liver Qi flowing smoothly and your liver functioning in harmony with its four other major partner organs, you can enjoy good health.
- The heart is the "king" of all the organs and houses a person's *Shen* or spirit.
- The spleen and stomach have an important partnership whereby the stomach receives food and liquid then the spleen transforms these elements into Acquired Qi that your whole body uses for nourishment and strength.
- From its high position in the chest, your lung governs both the formation of Qi, which occurs within the lung, and its distribution throughout the body.
- The kidney is the body's source of original Inborn Qi. It is responsible for a complex of functions including immune, sexual, and reproductive. As such, along with the liver, it plays a vital role in women's health.

PART TWO

GETTING TO THE ROOT CAUSE

CHAPTER 7

PERIMENOPAUSE:
Early Energy Signs and Symptoms of Imbalances That You Should Always Take Seriously

For most women, menopause comes on gradually over several years, in many cases over about a decade. The earliest stage is known in Western medicine as perimenopause. This is the time when your body is preparing for menopause.

In a perfect world, the perfect woman would make an easy, problem-free transition into menopause. She would be busy, but there would be a certain calmness about her, a certain peacefulness. Stress wouldn't bother her, and if she began to feel "out of sorts," she would take immediate action to improve her lifestyle with Taiji, yoga, or other gentle physical activity. She would know which foods to eat for energy and healing. She would never have had menstrual problems because her perfect body would have been functioning perfectly for many years! She would reach perimenopause around the age of forty-nine (when her seventh life cycle was complete). She wouldn't experience any negative symptoms and over a short time—maybe less than six months—the frequency of her periods would lessen until finally, one day (within a year), her periods would completely cease.

For most women, this perfect world is definitely not reality. Generally during perimenopause, you still have your monthly periods, and the process itself usually begins three to five years before your period ends. Perimenopause often starts when women are between the ages of forty-two to forty-five. The reason it starts earlier than our perfect woman? I believe there are three causes: stress, lifestyle, and eating habits. The most critical factor is stress.

In the real world, perimenopause is a time of natural transition. A woman's kidney Qi is beginning to decline as a result of growing older. (No one escapes growing older!) One by one, the Qi of each of her other organs is beginning to decline as well. Which organ falls out of balance first depends on which one's Qi is weakest. For most women this will be the liver—the organ that controls the menstrual cycle. It also is likely to be the spleen. Regardless of which organ changes first, the others will follow. Communications among them will, over time, begin to break down.

I often liken this process to a large corporation when a department supervisor retires and a new person arrives on the scene who does not have a good relationship with the other department heads. As a result, there will be infighting and competition, causing disarray in the whole organization, despite the fact that neither the company itself nor its president have changed.

SIGNS THAT PERIMENOPAUSE HAS BEGUN

As I've said, you are lucky because you are a woman. Your monthly menstrual cycle gives you signs to help you understand how your internal systems are doing. Instinctively, you learn to know if you are healthy. You are also lucky because menstruation is nature's own tune-up. With each monthly period, if your body is healthy, you have a unique opportunity to readjust it. If, on the other hand, you have difficulty with your menstrual cycle, your body is signaling you that your monthly internal tune-up process is not going smoothly. What if you've made a practice of continually masking various problems (such as menstrual cramps, headaches, PMS, and more that indicate deeper issues) when you were younger? You can almost count on these problems reemerging as more serious ones during the perimenopausal stage. Unfortunately for you, they didn't go away, they were just covered up. This is something I must really emphasize to my Western women patients: Healthy bodies do not have difficult menstrual cycles. Western women are so conditioned to suppress or cover up menstrual cycle problems that I spend a good deal of time helping them break through this mind-set.

During the perimenopausal transition then, it is not surprising that many women suffer from a wide variety of menstrual disorders. The following common problems all indicate a liver function disorder: PMS, mood swings, vaginal discharge, excessive bleeding, spotting, and irregular periods. Other symptoms might include urination frequency, weakness in the knees, cold hands and feet, constipation, sciatic pain, and lower back pain. Through my work with many Western women and their health problems, I have discovered that stress is the major external factor that causes a liver function disorder. If you suffer from these conditions, seek help at once and get yourself back into balance as quickly as possible. A lot of the advice that is in the chapters on self-healing can help you get on this path.

More often than not, when most women come to see me for perimenopausal conditions, I tell them that it's critical to address these problems today so that they can avoid a difficult menopause tomorrow. Let me show you what I mean.

Brenda was forty-seven when she first came to see me. She was a school teacher and mother of two teenage children. At the time, she still had her period and came to see me because of constipation and sciatic pain. I treated Brenda for both of these problems and was able to relieve these conditions. Besides the problems that caused her to come to me, a liver function disorder showed up when I performed her pulse diagnosis. So I warned her about the toll that stress was taking on her kidney and liver function. I told her that unless she started dealing with her perimenopausal issues, she would be back. Brenda stopped seeing me and I assume she continued her life in the way she always had because exactly two years later, she was back in my office.

But this time she had new symptoms. She was experiencing

major bleeding during her period, hot flashes every hour, and night sweats. Brenda's gynecologist wanted to put her on HRT. This frightened her, so she came back to see me first.

From her examination, I could tell that her kidney and liver function had gotten worse since we first met. So I gave her one of my classical herbal formulas in capsule. I told her that generally speaking, excessive bleeding is related to a Qi deficiency. This often occurs when women reach perimenopause because their bodies have just started to make this transition. The purpose of the herbs was to strengthen her overall Qi. She came back to see me twice, happy that the bleeding had completely stopped and her hot flashes and night sweats had disappeared. On her final visit, I again warned her that it was important to continue working on healing her kidney function by changing her diet and eating foods that would help strengthen this powerful organ. I told her that only her symptoms were under control, and if we stopped now, she would continue to lose Qi and that she could get a lot worse. Because Brenda found it almost impossible to change her lifestyle, I could tell she was a prime candidate for a serious kidney Qi deficiency. I recommended that she continue to see me for monthly acupuncture and herbs. I told her this would help her go through menopause smoothly.

But Brenda didn't come back until three months later when her hot flashes returned. Again I treated her and she improved. About six months later, Brenda returned, this time she had ringing in her ears. As we've seen, TCM considers the ear as the "window" of the kidney. So I knew immediately that Brenda's problem had progressed, and now, she did indeed have the condition about which I warned her—a serious kidney Qi deficiency.

From her history of problems, Brenda was finally beginning to realize that she needed to take responsibility for her own health and healing. This time she told me that she was committed to working together and that she wanted to make the necessary changes in her daily life and would take what I call "serious herbs," that is a special combination made just for her from the many dried herbal ingredients in my office. After two weeks of herbs, Brenda's hot flashes and ringing disappeared. She continued treatment for another two weeks and now comes in regularly for a tune-up. Finally understanding that she was responsible for her own health and healing, Brenda began to make tremendous strides in changing her lifestyle and diet. Her decision to put her health first and the demands of her very busy life a distant second was a real turning point.

I think many readers may relate to the kind of person that Brenda is. Before she made the changes in her life, she was the type of person who always has to finish something no matter how tired she was. She was the kind of person who would come home after work and could not go to bed before she cleaned her house. Her life was run by the clock. She had so many places to be and so many places to go. She continually told herself that she had to accomplish certain things—or else. She couldn't really tell me what would happen if she couldn't keep going, but her vague fears kept driving her onward. She could never sit still for any length of time. She continually pushed herself beyond her physical limits and ignored anything her body had to tell her.

Even if she was exhausted, she felt she had to work out. She could never really relax. In our early meetings, she continually asked me to tell her what the best things to do, or what the best Chinese pills were to "boost" her energy. One day I told her I had created a special recipe for her. I told her "Take one glass of champagne in a nice hot bath, light a candle, and listen to classical music. Then go to bed and have a nice sleep. I guarantee when you wake up you will have tremendous energy." I think she thought I was making a joke. When she would ask me these things, I always told her the best way to increase her energy was: "Do nothing!" I try to help all my patients to learn that "doing nothing" is actually "doing something." She never believed me until she finally decided to change herself. She now tells me how grateful she is to have learned to relax. Now, she can sit on her couch and sip a cup of tea while listening to classical music and get the same feeling (and the same benefits) she did when she finished her gym routine.

Today, I'm pleased to say Brenda is a healthy and happy

woman who has more energy than she ever dreamed possible. She was most skeptical about making lifestyle changes. Why? Because she just couldn't believe that stress was actually damaging her physical body. Sure, she knew it made her a little "nuts" as she put it, but she didn't recognize stress for the destructive agent that it is. Many of my menopause patients are like Brenda. Once they decide to help themselves, they become so happy. I know that you can do the same thing for yourself as well.

EXCESSIVE BLEEDING: WESTERN AND EASTERN SOLUTIONS

Many women come to me with complaints of excessive bleeding, one of the most common symptoms of perimenopause. Some have very long periods or might menstruate twice within a single month. From the TCM point of view, what is happening is that their Qi is declining and weakening. It can no longer do its job of controlling the blood. Remember what I said about Qi being the "commander" of blood, and blood being the "mother" of Qi? This relationship, of course, is especially important for women; when you lose blood during your period, you lose Qi as well. Excessive bleeding drains the body's Qi, so it's very important to strengthen Qi and get the blood back under control. Ginseng is one herb that can help. When a woman is bleeding excessively, this is one of the rare times I recommend taking it. (There are healing recipes with ginseng in Chapter 14.) When there is excessive bleeding, it is essential to treat the liver as well.

Western and Eastern medicine have very different points of view in this regard. If a woman is suffering from severe menstrual disorders such as excessive bleeding during perimenopause, Western doctors often recommend surgery in the belief that the simplest and most effective solution is to remove the uterus or ovaries, or both. An added argument is that this surgical procedure can also reduce the risk of uterine cancer.

It appears that women are taking this advice in record numbers. There has been a dramatic increase in hysterectomies in recent years. In fact, it is now one of the most performed surgical procedures in the United States. One out of four women in the United States is plunged into menopause artificially and prematurely by surgery.

TCM does not regard this procedure as a desirable one under most circumstances. In addition to an abrupt menopause, a hysterectomy can bring in its wake a host of problems, both physical and emotional. They include: prolapse (the falling) of the other abdominal organs, constipation, lower back pain, osteoporosis, sexual and urinary problems, chronic fatigue, depression, and increased risk of heart disease. Even Western medicine acknowledges that some women suffer more after a hysterectomy than before. Additionally, a hysterectomy leaves no option for the many women who are postponing childbirth until their later years.

I would like women to discover that there are indeed other options. But, why do many more women choose the Western path? I think I understand why. Quite often, heavy bleeding can be extremely frightening for a woman. Seeking advice, she turns to the person she knows and trusts—her OB/GYN. If she is experiencing a great deal of discomfort or stress about her situation, the last thing she feels inclined to do is search for other opinions. At this time, she has neither the physical or mental stamina to handle this effort. The truth is, however, this is the most important time to seek another viewpoint. Many of my patients come to see me when everything else has failed, often when their conditions have gone from good to bad, or bad to worse.

As I've said before, Western medicine tends to see a woman's reproductive organs as expendable after menopause. In other words, the uterus and ovaries are physical structures that are no longer needed. The TCM view, as you know by now, is quite different. Think of how powerful your uterus is. It has enough Qi to actually create and sustain the life force of another human being. TCM categorizes the uterus as an "extra" organ. It is very reluctant to remove this "extra" organ (or any other organ, for that matter).

Removing an organ disrupts the energetic unity and balance of the body irrevocably, and makes real healing on a fundamental level much more difficult. Even after the childbearing years are over, a woman's uterus is still animated by Qi, and connected via the meridians with the body's whole energy system. It is still "part of the family." Given the proper support, the uterus is still able to perform its function, and, as I've said many times throughout this book, help your body produce enough hormones for the rest of your life. It is fair to say that Western medicine has not yet developed an understanding of this vital Qi connection and that reproductive organs still carry "messages" for the rest of the body.

One of my patients, Judy, who was forty-five when she came to see me, had never had menstrual problems and considered herself very healthy. During the previous six months her lifestyle had gotten quite crazy. She was traveling far more than she ever had. Her job had gotten increasingly demanding. She and her husband had built a new house and she was expecting her mother-in-law to move in. Inside, she was aware that something had changed. For the first time ever during her menstrual cycle, she had pain and bright red bleeding. Her period was two to three days late, and she was spotting in the middle of her menstrual cycle. She said that during the holidays, she bled more than she ever had before, which frightened her. Her OB/GYN said if things didn't improve, she might want to consider surgery.

I told Judy that what she was experiencing was "normal." I explained how many women who reach this transitional time in their lives find that their menstrual cycle changes. However, I said that the symptoms could get worse unless we did something now. So I taught her Qigong movements, made suggestions about healing foods she could add to her diet, gave her herbs to help improve her liver function, and made several strong recommendations about lifestyle areas she needed to change if she didn't want to see this condition worsen. Because she arrived in my office as a very healthy woman, I only needed to see her for about three weeks. After this, her excessive bleeding stopped. Also, she was a disciplined individual and a very good student. She immediately began to incorporate all the things I recommended. Now, Judy comes to me about twice a year for a TCM tune-up. There is no need for any additional treatment. I do not expect her to have a difficult menopause. Neither she nor I expect that she will need to take hormones.

WHAT TCM DOES FOR PERIMENOPAUSE

My own approach to perimenopause is as follows:

Step 1 is to create harmony among the patient's organs. It's very important to try to get a woman's whole energy system back on line and in balance during the early stages of menopause, because I know from experience that later it will be much more difficult, and she will suffer even more from menopausal symptoms.

During perimenopause, most women's Qi needs a general "tonifying" and strengthening—in other words, an overall tune-up. This has to be done before I can begin treating specific organs. It's as if her whole body is behind a cloud—it's hard to see clearly and more difficult for me to see the root cause of her particular problem. So I have to wait and try to balance the whole body first before I begin a deeper treatment.

At this point, if symptoms are mild, I usually give my patients one or two kinds of classical herbal formulas, *Xiao Chai Hu Tang* and *Liu Wei Di Huang Wan*, which can be found in almost any Chinese food market. With these herbs, they almost always experience immediate benefits. Their constipation ends, which causes the wrinkles around their eyes to disappear, and they see positive changes in their menstrual cycles. Inside their bodies, the communications between their organs starts to improve. And that is very good news for both of us. If they are under a lot of stress and exhibit more severe symptoms, then I will give patients my own formulas, which are based on ancient, classical formulas. I have adapted these for the Western lifestyle; they are called *Green Dragon,* which helps improve liver function and *Imperial Qi,* which helps strengthen kidney Qi.

Step 2 is to help women rebalance their emotions. Remember emotions have a very powerful effect on your body and can do a lot either to support or undermine your healing process. In my opinion, Western women get very little emotional support, especially as they grow older. They are constantly bombarded with negative messages and difficult choices they are forced to consider, which engender fear about growing older, becoming ill, or having a disease.

Women rarely receive positive, hopeful uplifting messages about their own healing power and abilities at this time. Their attention is directed toward fear and loss and potential health risks and problems. Seldom are they told that menopause is a deeply enriching time and one of spiritual expansion.

That's why at this stage, I try to help my patients understand that this transition can be a very real gift and perhaps the best opportunity for change they've ever been given. I help them learn how to use the power of their thoughts to improve their health and their lives. This step is an essential part of treatment. It is not just "happy talk;" it is my job to create a positive environment within which my women patients can unlock their own healing abilities.

When we talk, I often get them to smile and even laugh. Each individual is different. Sometimes I create a story that helps illustrate what I want them to learn, and this too often ends up making them laugh. When they leave my office, they have usually left a lot of stress behind and feel more positive and more confident in their own power.

Many times I make a joke and say, "Next time you come you should bring a big plastic bag." When they ask me why, I tell them: "It's for all the garbage you've left behind!" When I get my patients to smile, I am actually practicing the highest form of ancient Chinese medicine. If I can help them to smile from their hearts (which they often do), then, their heart, the "king of all the organs," will help stimulate their Qi and its companion blood to flow more freely among their organs and throughout their body. This helps open a door inside them and can begin a special healing process. Smiling and laughing have a profound effect on the material body.

I remind my patients, even as I remind you, that when it comes to emotions, the liver is exceptionally vulnerable to anger, stress, and depression. These emotions, if experienced chronically, will affect the way the liver performs its many essential functions. When a woman experiences a liver function disorder, all her symptoms are aggravated. I encourage my patients (and you as well) to do everything within their power to reduce the stress in their lives and nurture themselves so that they have a more calm and peaceful mind. I teach them the unique Qigong movements that you will find in Chapter 13. These have the special power to unite your body, mind, and spirit. They also offer a powerful way to conserve Qi as well.

Step 3 is to educate my patients about how to conserve Qi. Conserving Qi is always important, especially as we grow older. I advise my patients not to overwork, to rest more frequently, and to try to keep to a regular schedule. This will help them to stabilize their Qi during this time of change. I also tell them not to exercise too much, and to replace strenuous exercises such as jogging or aerobics with "soft" exercise like yoga, Taiji, or swimming. Certain foods are also particularly good to strengthen a woman's Qi, especially sour pickles, onions, scallions, rosemary, and ginger (see Recipes for Healing). These foods generally support kidney and liver Qi.

The principles behind TCM treatment during perimenopause are:

- Address the problem before it becomes more serious;
- Fix the urgent problems first; then find and fix their root cause;
- Try to prevent any new problems from arising.

Remember, TCM concerns itself not only with presenting problems, but with what happened in the past to cause them and what might happen in the future if they aren't healed at the source. If you listen to and respond to your body's signals, especially during perimenopause, then according to TCM, your transition through menopause will be shorter and easier. In other words, your body will need less time to go through change and this change can actually benefit your body, mind, and spirit.

In the next chapter, let's look at the many symptoms women experience when they are in full-blown menopause.

TO SUMMARIZE:

- Perimenopause is the first stage of menopause, or what TCM calls "Menstrual Cycle Ending Symptoms."
- For most women, it begins between ages forty-two and forty-five, about three to five years before menstruation ends.
- In a perfect world, perimenopause should begin at age forty-nine, when a woman's seventh life cycle ends. But for many women, the stresses of modern life have caused it to begin earlier.
- During perimenopause, a woman's internal Qi is starting to decline, and one by one the function of her organs is beginning to slow down or perform poorly. Which organ changes first depends on which is weakest. For virtually everyone—men and women— it's the kidney.
- Among the most common symptoms experienced during perimenopause are PMS, mood swings, vaginal discharge, excessive bleeding, spotting, irregular periods, urinary frequency, knee weakness, cold hands and feet, constipation, sciatic pain, and lower back pain.
- My approach to treatment is creating harmony, controlling emotions, and conserving Qi.
- I also try to catch the problem before it becomes more serious; fix the urgent problems first; then find and fix their root cause; and try to prevent new problems from arising.

CHAPTER 8

MENOPAUSE:
Being in the Heart of It

*B*ASED on my experience with thousands of Western women, I can tell you that most of them regard the passage through menopause as anything but natural. But one of the root causes of menopause is very natural. A kidney Qi deficiency is part of the natural law. All living things have a cycle of birth and death. Every one of us is going to lose kidney Qi—that's what constitutes the aging process. You have no control over whether or not you're born with a lot of kidney Qi or a little. Remember that the ancient Chinese believed that in life's lottery you may receive a short candle or a tall one; how you take care of its flame is up to you.

In the same way, the quantity of your life may be out of your hands, but controlling its quality is up to you. You very definitely have control over keeping your liver healthy. And now you know why this is so important: TCM considers it the most important organ for women's health. If you create problems that affect your liver, they can be reversed. Like so many of the women I see, you may think you have no way out of your current lifestyle, but let me give you some serious food for thought. Your lifestyle can permanently destroy your health. Stress is the number one external factor impacting liver function; anger is the number one internal factor.

Look at how crazy our Western lifestyle has become. People are flooded with communications almost twenty-four hours a day. There are office faxes, home faxes, home phones with call waiting and caller ID, office phones connected to hundreds of other phones, car phones, web sites, home pages, beepers, and more. It's almost as if we're being programmed by something else. Some people literally cannot stop themselves during the day to take five minutes to close their eyes and meditate so that that can rejuvenate themselves. This is not right. In fact, I tell my patients that the world is really upside down. We should be resting and meditating or practicing Qigong a lot more, not squeezing these things in.

One of my male patients wears three beepers, carries two cellular phones, and works from three Internet addresses. (Some of my women patients are only a little better.) This is bad for his health, whether he knows it or not. I'm afraid some of my women patients are also destroying their health in the same way. New communications techniques are controlling us; it should be the other way around. And they are contributing enormously to the stress in our lives. We should recognize this and take steps to reverse the problem. If you add up the other external stresses and some of the emotional issues we carry with us, you can see why when women reach the age of menopause, their bodies have become unbalanced. Now let's look at how these factors can influence the course of your menopause more closely.

With the onset of certain symptoms such as vaginal dryness, hot flashes, and night sweats, you have moved out of the early transitional phase and are fully into menopause. In addition to these three symptoms, other telltale signs that menopause has arrived include a loss of sex drive, urinary infections, abnormal mood swings, and a decrease in the frequency of monthly periods. Additional symptoms that might also occur are insomnia, digestive problems such as heartburn, as well as shortness of breath and heart palpitations. Western medicine considers the menopausal transition completed when no bleeding has occurred for one year.

Let's discuss each of these symptoms in more detail. You'll

begin to see how they are all related to the deeper root cause—almost always, from my experience with Western women—of a kidney Qi deficiency and a liver function disorder. Sometimes one or more of the other five major organs is involved. In the case of the kidney, menopausal symptoms can worsen in its related season, the winter. Consequently, you should be aware that symptoms related to kidney Qi deficiency like hot flashes are often more frequent during winter months.

HOT FLASHES AND NIGHT SWEATS

Laura is a designer of women's clothing. When she first came to see me, she was fifty years old. She was having a difficult menopause. She had hot flashes during the day and night sweats. Her stomach was totally distended; she suffered from headaches, which had been going on literally for years. In recent months, she had developed carpal tunnel syndrome. Laura initially came to see me because of the problem with her wrists.

The first thing we addressed was her carpal tunnel problem by treating it with acupuncture and acupressure. I told her that it was easy to treat her wrists, but that her problems would persist if she and I didn't also work on rebalancing or restoring normal liver function. TCM understands that tendons are the tissue or "sinew" of the liver and that all tendon problems are related to the liver. I also told her that like so many of my other Western women patients around her age, she was experiencing problems with her Qi. From my diagnosis, I could tell that her Qi deficiency was related to two major organs: the kidney and the spleen.

If the spleen is weak, the body can't requisition enough Qi for its daily mental and physical activities from food. If the kidney is weak, it doesn't have the power to support the body's overall functions. It's very important to strengthen these two organs because they constitute the body's main sources of Qi, or vital energy.

So Laura began to take classical herbs for her liver, kidney, and spleen. I prescribed several Qigong movements that she practiced regularly. Almost immediately her hot flashes and night sweats disappeared; this enabled her to sleep more soundly through the night. As her sleep improved, her body was able to generate a better healing "charge" during the night and use this time to repair itself naturally. I also recommended that she eat roasted walnuts every morning, eat as much seafood as possible to strengthen her kidney Qi, and gave her Chinese ginseng.

When Laura came to see me a few weeks later, her headaches were totally gone. When she asked me how this was possible, I told her that together we helped boost her overall energy system so that it could function again. Once this began to happen, her own organs took over the job of rebalancing themselves and healing her problems.

Gradually we were able to bring her spleen back in balance and now her stomach problems are also gone. Laura continues to come for regular "tune-ups" with acupuncture. But one of the best things about Laura's treatment is that she is committed to continue working by herself to maintain her balance. She even participated in my Dragon's Way® Program for weight loss and stress management and lost eight pounds!

Estimates are that more than 80 percent of women in menopause experience hot flashes. Hot flashes and night sweats are a good indicator that you have moved fully into menopause. With these conditions, your body cannot maintain its normal temperature range; it's become too hot and cannot cool itself off. Your declining kidney Qi is not strong enough to cool the fire of your heart, which has become excessive. Your liver is not functioning smoothly enough to promote the free flow of the body's Qi, so it's now become blocked and stagnant and it too generates heat.

When I talk about conditions of stagnation or internal heat, my Western patients are sometimes puzzled by these concepts. I compare Qi stagnation with the idea of a compost heap. Temperatures inside a compost heap can be so hot, you cannot thrust your hand too deeply inside or you can get burned. Flames may not be spewing from a compost heap, but nevertheless, it can generate very high temperatures. Even without any external heat source, the pressure and kinds of organic and inorganic matter inside a compost heap slowly cause a heat buildup.

When you're suffering from hot flashes or night sweats, your lung, whose job it is to distribute Qi and help regulate body temperature, also does not get sufficient support from the kidney. Thus, the lung doesn't have enough strength to command the body's Qi, and circulation becomes poor. The natural automatic transfer of Qi between the body's interior and exterior that is supposed to take place at the skin and cool your body then becomes impaired. The result is that heat begins to accumulate further and a hot flash occurs. For some women, these hot flashes or night sweats occur so frequently and so violently that they are debilitating. Please note that you can attempt to cool yourself off externally and you'll gain some relief, but if you want your hot flashes and night sweats to go away, you've got to address their internal root cause.

Often a woman will suffer more from heat and sweating either during the day or at night. This has to do with the body's balance of yin and yang Qi and which is weakest. In Chapter 3, we talked about these two types of Qi. Yang Qi is related to daytime, the sun, and heat. Yin Qi is cooler, and is related to the night and the moon. If you feel hot and perspire a lot during the day, it means your yang Qi is deficient. It is too weak to control the opening and closing of the pores. This impairs the release of sweat and interferes with the regulation of body temperature. Yang Qi deficiency is at the root of the familiar menopausal involuntary release of heat and sweat.

If you suffer more from night sweats, it means that your yin Qi is deficient. This deficiency results in too much heat inside the body. This condition is particularly aggravated at night when yang Qi follows its normal nocturnal course and moves from the body's surface to its interior. If you suffer equally from heat and sweating during the day and at night, both your yin and yang Qi are deficient. Because yin and yang Qi differ, so too will TCM treatment depending on which of them is deficient. In either case, the goal is to recharge your body's Qi. For these conditions, I like to say, "The radio is okay, it just needs a battery charge."

In addition to an energy recharge, at this time I use specific herbs and a course of acupuncture. Sometimes a month or so of treatment is all that's needed to eliminate symptoms and prevent their recurrence. I also emphasize to my patients the importance of "eating for energy" in the healing process. There is a great deal of self-healing a woman can do on her own if she knows the right foods to eat to support the Qi of various organs, especially the kidney, liver, and spleen. I've compiled a lot of this information for you in Chapter 15.

Let's return to our banking analogy for a moment: Remember you're born with a certain amount of Qi. This energy foundation comes from your parents and is stored in your kidney. You can consider this your Qi savings account, an account that we are drawing on from the minute we're born to support the function of all the organs. You can never get enough kidney Qi. After birth, we get most of our Qi from another source. This is the food we eat, which the spleen transforms into Qi as well. This forms our Qi checking account. This is the account we can and should add to, and this is the one from which we should be drawing for our daily Qi. With good quality foods, the spleen can produce new Qi continuously. The stronger it is, the less we have to draw upon the finite Qi of the kidney. The more we can save our kidney Qi, the longer and healthier our lives. This underscores the importance of eating well and good digestion.

The lung is also a major organ in the production of Qi. If your lung is weak, you may have more problems related to Qi deficiency, as well as symptoms such as asthma or a chronic cough.

MIND AND EMOTIONS

TCM believes that the body and mind are inseparable, and cannot be treated in isolation from one another. A good TCM doctor also has to be a good psychologist. According to the ancient Five Element Theory, each of the five major organs in the body—liver, heart, spleen, lung, and kidney—responds to and is affected by a different emotion. It's as if these emotions are like tuning forks that vibrate at the same frequency as the organs. Things are fine as long as everything is in balance. The heart, for instance, corresponds with happiness, and needs to feel peaceful and relaxed in order to function well. Problems in the organs will affect our emotions and, to an even greater degree, our emotions will affect our organs. Every organ needs a certain amount of Qi to fuel its function, and it also needs the right message to guide that function, like a computer program. Excess emotion is a kind of out-of-control Qi that can impair an organ's function by disrupting its normal programming.

And which emotion relates to the liver's health? Of course, you now know it's anger. Chronic anger is the single most destructive internal force capable of disrupting, or even destroying, liver function; stress is the single most destructive external force. Remember that this is the organ whose main principle is that of free flow. The liver likes and *needs* to feel smooth and relaxed. If you're not, it's not.

This information is especially critical for women. The liver is very susceptible to problems of stagnation caused by the corresponding emotions mentioned above: anger, stress, and depression. All of these, especially stress, have a negative effect on liver Qi. If the liver is out of order, it will affect your whole body's circulation, and thus every other organ. Think about what stagnation can mean to your menstrual cycle and the smooth flow of blood. This is a dynamic to which you should always pay careful attention; nothing in your body happens in isolation.

When a woman reaches menopause, not only is her physical Qi lower than it was when she was younger, but her whole body is in a state of change. At the same time, between job and family she often has more responsibility than ever. Thus, her life is sometimes at its most stressful just when she needs to be most relaxed and calm.

A calm state is not easy to achieve—you have to make every

effort to manage your daily life, and to change yourself. Many things outside of us cannot be changed; the demands of work and family cannot simply be ignored. You can, however, change yourself: by changing daily habits, controlling emotions, managing stress, and developing new attitudes. In the section of this book on self-healing I've outlined many ways you can change your daily life, increase Qi, and become more peaceful. The most important thing is to keep your thinking positive. Don't think you are sick—you are not sick. Your body is in a state of transition. Your organs (both their physiological and psychological aspects) are just not functioning well, and they are not communicating with each other. This can cause a great deal of discomfort, but it is not a disease.

A lot of menopausal women suffer from feelings of irritability, anger, even rage, depression, and nervousness, all of which have to do with poor liver function.

Insomnia is also common. Night sweats are one major cause of sleeplessness; poor digestion is another. Because the body's Qi is weak, it has more trouble processing food. The same holds true of emotions. The worries and stresses of the day tend to get stuck in your body and accumulate, disrupting sleep and causing bad dreams, so that you wake up as tired as when you went to bed. It's a vicious cycle. And the most powerful healing thing you can do for yourself is to break this cycle.

One of the most distressing emotions that women may experience during and after menopause is depression. Some women get so depressed that they feel immobilized, and they turn to antidepressants to help them cope. But these drugs don't heal or rebalance depressed feelings; they just cover them up. You may no longer be as aware of it, but the feeling is still there. Under the surface, emotions are cooking, and heat is rising. You never know when this volcano might erupt, and if it does, there will be no way to control it. As with all drugs, antidepressants only drive the problem deeper into the body. They also make the body dependent on help from the outside, so that later you may have even more problems.

When you undergo a major transition, like menopause, your body and mind literally can't work together. Drugs can look like a real solution, and they may be—temporarily. When you're feeling so depressed that it's hard to function, you may think that you just can't make it on your own. But if you want to truly get better, you have to fight, there's no easy way. Think about it. Can you rely on these drugs for the long-term? If you stop taking them and you still feel bad, what then? Can your body tolerate them forever? If you go off your antidepressants and your problems resurface, it means that the drugs were only covering them up.

From my experience with helping Western women with depression, I've learned a lot. One of my patients had been suffering from depression and been on medication for twenty-five years. I treated the root cause of her condition for several months. Usually, depression relates to the relationship between the liver and the spleen. Little by little, I was able to help her see that she had the skill and ability to heal this condition. We talked about how her whole body was out of balance. I didn't tell her to stop taking her medication; as her organs came back into balance, her own body told her to stop. When her body began to work in harmony for the first time in a long time, she felt healthy. She worked with her Western doctor to lower her dosage. Finally, she was able to stop all medication.

Another patient in her mid-forties returned to me several times because of fibroid tumors in her uterus. She was deeply depressed because of their return and convinced that her next step would have to be a hysterectomy. Again, we worked at healing the root cause of this problem and talked of the many ways this woman could use her own healing ability to help herself.

My youngest case of depression was a nine-year-old boy who had been to several psychiatrists and was being given antidepressants, which were causing severe side effects. How could someone so young have this kind of problem? While many children might dislike going to school, for this young boy it produced acute problems. His condition was so bad that he could not go to school because he would suffer from such severe stomachaches that he would have to be sent home. His psychiatrist referred him to me for whatever help I could give. Again, I treated the root cause and his problem gradually disappeared.

If you suffer from depression, my advice to you is not to give up. Try to find a skilled acupuncturist and TCM doctor who can work with you to heal the root cause of your condition. Be patient. Work with your Western doctor and be sure and tell him or her what you are doing so that you are supported in your efforts to add complementary medicine to your healing tools.

Suppressing problems of depression rather than healing them at the root is like trying to hold a ball under water. When there's just one ball, you can hold it down with one hand. If another ball appears, you'll have to use both hands. But what if a third ball pops to the surface, and a fourth? You're never going to be able to keep them all under water, and you'll only exhaust yourself trying. To heal for real, you must alleviate the cause. That's why TCM will try to fix the body's weakest point at the root, before the problem goes deeper and spreads to other organs. Rather than giving you a cane on which to lean, (that might well break some day), TCM strengthens the whole body, so that you can support yourself. Particularly when it comes to the emotions, you have to learn to deal with them on your own. If I help my patients too much with their emotions, they'll never be able to do this job for themselves.

DIGESTIVE PROBLEMS

During menopause, none of the organs are functioning very well, and the whole body's Qi is low. One common way this situation manifests itself is in digestive problems. Digestion is slower and less efficient, and the body tends to hold on to water and fat. Many menopausal women suffer from either constipation or diarrhea, abdominal distention, indigestion, and nausea. They tend to gain weight, and may begin to have food allergies they never had before. They may not be able to eat the amount or kinds of foods they could when they were younger; things that never used to be a problem affect them differently now.

Why is this? Western tests would probably show nothing wrong physiologically with their stomachs or any other organ. The problem is not physical, the problem is functional. TCM has a complete theoretical framework for recognizing and treating poor organ function. In this case, the two major organs involved are the kidney and the liver, especially the liver. In my experience, Western lifestyle is responsible for 90 percent of digestive problems, which are caused by poor liver function. Although the spleen—the major organ of digestion—suffers, it is not the root cause.

In the Five Element Theory, wood (the liver) controls earth (the spleen). The spleen depends upon the support and regulation of the liver. Thus, good liver function is critical to the process of digestion. Liver Qi must be strong and smooth, which it seldom is in women with a stressful lifestyle. Many menopausal women are caught in a cycle of increasing stress. At the very time they are undergoing a major energetic and physical transition, they also find themselves coping with substantial external pressures—pressure from the job, pressure from their family, pressure from their many obligations—which make them more nervous, which in turn creates more stress. So many of my patients are simultaneously dealing with one or more serious issues, including their own lifestyle changes, their children leaving home permanently, moving their job or their home, divorce, retirement issues, the death of a spouse, the care or death of a parent. It's amazing that their bodies and spirits can withstand so much. Add to this the fact that they may not be eating or sleeping well. It is not surprising at all that the Qi they need to heal themselves is not being recharged. This harmful cycle must be reversed for a woman's liver and digestive system to function well.

Here's a true story that illustrates how and why lifestyle plays such a major role in menopausal symptoms. I have one patient who is an artist. She came to me for hot flashes and night sweats. These were so bad that they were disrupting her life. She was very reluctant to begin HRT, although some of her doctors had already recommended that she start.

Her friend had recommended that she see me. We had a very lucky relationship. She took several of my classical herbal formulas and after two weeks, her symptoms abated by about 80 percent, which given their severity, really surprised her. I told her that her body was very sensitive to energy or Qi and that she could benefit enormously from learning one simple Qigong exercise, which I taught her. Like many ancient TCM doctors, I used this Qigong movement like a prescription. It helped her unite her body and spirit. She became calmer and more peaceful. We continued our appointments for several more weeks. She reported that her symptoms were about 90 percent gone. Now, she could recognize that her hot flashes and night sweats were directly related to her stress level. If she painted well, she could feel that her day went very well and that she didn't have her menopausal problems. Little by little she began to understand how stress was directly affecting her overall well-being. For two more months, she took the classical herbs and all symptoms disappeared.

Eight months later though, she returned because her hot flashes had returned. What happened? She told me her son had lost his job and had moved in with her. Unfortunately, they fought all the time. Her family situation caused renewed stress, high blood pressure, migraine headaches, and more discomforts than before. Even though she could recognize the root cause of her current conditions, the problems had come on so suddenly and so acutely that they had gone too far for her to help herself. Once again, we went through a series of treatments that helped her regain her internal balance. Now, more than ever, she also recognized the power of Qigong and began practicing every day. I tell you this story to point out that even though something can be 100 percent fixed, you can still reactivate the problems if conditions are right. Watch your lifestyle carefully so you can avoid recurring health issues.

Here's another case study. A very successful saleswoman

came to me complaining of sleep disturbances, hot flashes, and night sweats. Because her family had a history of breast cancer, she too was reluctant to begin HRT. She wanted to work with TCM first to treat her problem. She had been my patient for several years before her menopause and she was also a Qigong student in my school. When we used herbs and Qigong, all her symptoms were completely eliminated. I warned her that she had to protect and conserve her Qi if she didn't want them to return. Then she got a big new job. You can guess what happened. She threw herself into this new situation. She began to eat poorly, her digestion system became weak, then her energy declined, and her hot flashes returned. A few months later, she returned with more symptoms. She had just become the volunteer president of her women's club. She had more jobs and more worries than she knew what to do with. Each of them consumed more of her mental, spiritual, emotional, and physical resources. Now, even the herbs could not help her because she pushed herself beyond her body's natural healthy capacity for her stage of life. We both worked for a long time to rebalance her entire energy system. Please pay attention to the demands of your own lifestyle. Here's an area of responsibility where you do have a lot of control.

Don't question your healing ability if your menopausal symptoms return. Don't question the usefulness of working with your TCM doctor. Don't wonder if your herbs are powerful enough. If your symptoms recur, it is normally because you have experienced a lifestyle or emotional change that has exceeded the current limits of your body's level of Qi. The answers lie within you. The answers lie in examining where and how your lifestyle is draining your Qi and figuring out how to save it.

When it comes to healthy digestion, both the liver and the spleen need the support of a strong kidney. Any treatment of digestive problems has to improve the function of all of these organs, especially the liver. TCM herbs can help. But food is better than herbs: you have to learn what to eat. You also have to learn how to eat in a way that supports the function of your digestive system. We'll cover all of this in Chapter 15.

VAGINAL DRYNESS, LOSS OF SEX DRIVE, AND URINARY INFECTIONS

As a woman ages, the walls of the vagina become thinner, dryer, less elastic, and more vulnerable to infection. The vagina also shrinks, becoming progressively shorter and narrower. Symptoms of vaginal atrophy such as irritation, burning, and lack of lubrication during sex can be one of the first signs of menopause. These symptoms can cause distress and discomfort at any time, but they can have a deeper effect on a woman's sex life as intercourse becomes uncomfortable or even painful. She may also be more susceptible to vaginal infections after sex. At the same time, a woman may be experiencing a loss of sex drive. Western medicine explains all this as due to a drop in hormone levels. Hormone levels are dropping—but why? TCM also understands that the hormone levels are dropping, but it pursues this further by searching for the root cause. If you are healthy, you can look back and see that your hormones weren't dropping when you were twenty years old, were they? Or thirty? What happened? TCM traces this, of course, to your kidney, the body's Qi foundation. TCM believes that the kidney controls the whole endocrine system. When kidney Qi decreases, as a consequence, hormone levels drop. That's why TCM always treats endocrine problems by treating the kidney first. Once again, remember the physical organ itself may appear perfectly fine; tests of the organ may be normal. We are describing the complex of functions that relate to the kidney. According to TCM, when hormone levels drop, the kidney is definitely not functioning at its best.

Because the liver meridians encircle the genitals, deficient liver Qi also plays a part in reducing sexual desire (as does age; diminishing sexual drive is in part a natural process). In the TCM view, the only way to deal with these problems at the source is to strengthen kidney Qi, not an easy thing to do. Herbs can help, as can certain foods that support both the kidney and the liver (see Chapter 15). Practicing *Wu Ming* Meridian Therapy can help the most.

Lack of kidney Qi is also at the root of changes in the tissues of the urinary tract, and symptoms such as incontinence and urinary infections. In TCM, the kidney and bladder share a very close relationship, like brother and sister. They communicate or send messages back and forth through Qi. For instance, the kidney tells the bladder to hold all urine until morning. These are instantaneous, automatic messages that flow smoothly back and forth between the organs when you are healthy. Antibiotics are often prescribed for urinary tract infections, but these infections tend to recur, leading to long-term drug use. TCM does not see them as real "infections," but as a problem of Qi stagnation. TCM treatment will try not only to strengthen kidney function, but try to make both kidney and bladder Qi flow more smoothly.

While it's important as always to try to heal the root cause, herbs can bring fast relief from the discomfort of both urinary tract and vaginal infections. Temporary relief from symptoms such as vaginal irritation, burning, and dryness can also be found in natural lubricants, such as pure *Aloe vera* gel. Try to avoid petroleum products, which tend to be allergenic and difficult for the body to process. Estrogen creams can be used locally to restore vaginal secretions and tissue elasticity, but you may run some of the same cancer risks with these vaginal creams as with oral estrogens.

To help heal yourself, it is vital to bring as much calm as possible into your life. Now you know why this isn't just a nice admonition. Peace and calm can bring direct benefits to the health of your liver and other organs. Perhaps you've already discovered that a calm state is not easy to achieve. But you should make every effort to manage your daily life, change yourself, and take time out to care for yourself. These are not selfish things to do; these are self-healing things to do. Do it now, do it for yourself and the people you love, do not wait until later. Remember that you are always in control of the ability to change from within. And not only can you change yourself, but you can also heal yourself. Here are a few suggestions:

- Really look at your daily lifestyle and determine where you can make healthy changes in your daily habits;
- Learn what triggers any emotional outbursts;
- Try changing things that trigger emotional shifts;
- Find ways to manage stress (practicing relaxation exercises, yoga, Taiji, Qigong, noncompetitive swimming);
- Develop new attitudes, new interests; avoid taking on too many obligations that you alone must meet;
- Teach yourself to let go of emotions and things;
- Do less; rest more.

Remember menopause is not a disease. I hope the ancient wisdom in this book will give you a new perspective and help you achieve a larger degree of control over any menopausal symptoms you may be struggling with. Helping yourself through this natural transition and using the time-tested principles, theories, techniques, and tools of TCM will allow your body to produce enough hormones to last a lifetime!

PALPITATIONS AND SHORTNESS OF BREATH

Sometimes during menopause, women may experience palpitations or shortness of breath. If they go shopping, they may feel fatigued. If they go up and down steps, they may experience shortness of breath. They may not be able to chase their grandchild as easily as they used to. The root cause of this kind of condition is kidney Qi deficiency.

Palpitations are a results of a disruption in the relationship between the kidney and the heart. Kidney Qi deficiency has caused the heart's Qi to become weak. This is a classical TCM example of "Water and Fire Cannot Achieve Harmony." The kidney cannot control the heart so you experience palpitations. Often women become very alarmed at this symptom because they are aware of the fact that heart disease is their number one killer.

Shortness of breath, from the TCM perspective, is a result of an imbalance between the kidney and the lung, or the kidney and the heart. When kidney Qi deficiency develops, the kidney acts like a petty thief and robs Qi from the lung. This is a classical TCM example of "The 'Child' Steals Qi from its 'Mother'." With all of these symptoms, you can begin to appreciate how important it is to keep kidney Qi strong during the transition of menopause. You can also begin to see why all these seemingly unconnected conditions actually have only one root cause.

NATURAL MENOPAUSE VERSUS CHEMICAL OR SURGICAL MENOPAUSE: COMBATING THE SYMPTOMS

After Cesarean sections, hysterectomies (removal of the uterus) are the second most-performed procedure on women in the United States. One source states that by the age of sixty, one third of American women will have had hysterectomies. Other studies suggest this rate is higher. If the ovaries are removed, this procedure is called an oophorectomy. When ovaries are removed in a premenopausal woman, her body will be abruptly thrown into menopause with its attendant symptoms. TCM considers this menopause different from a naturally occurring one. And because the cause is different, the treatment will be different as well.

Some women enter menopause naturally and others become menopausal through surgery. Today there is still a third cause of menopause: drugs such as tamoxifen. Tamoxifen is an antiestrogenic agent that was first approved by the FDA for use in breast cancer treatment in 1977. Following this development, tamoxifen was used to treat early and advanced stage breast cancer. In 1992, in what has turned out to be a landmark study, The Breast Cancer Prevention Trial (BCPT), was launched to evaluate tamoxifen as a breast cancer preventive agent. A total of 13, 388 women participated. In April 1998, breast cancer researchers announced that tamoxifen had been found to reduce breast cancer cases by 45 percent in women at high risk for the disease. At that time, federal health experts estimated that more than 21 million women could be eligible for tamoxifen therapy.

Let's look at how tamoxifen works. Researchers describe its mechanism of action like this: "Tamoxifen works by interfering with the interaction of breast cancer cells and estrogen, a hormone involved in the division and growth of cancerous cells. Tamoxifen attaches to the receptor in the cells and 'sees' estrogen and prevents the cell from 'seeing' estrogen. So, it can actually stop the growth of breast cells and breast cancer cells."

Unfortunately, for many women with breast cancer, tamoxifen has also proven to have certain side effects. The BCPT study cites the increased risk of uterine cancer and blood clots traveling from the legs to the lungs. There are a number of other studies that have tracked critical, although less dramatic, side effects. Some side effects, notably hot flashes, have been debilitating enough to cause withdrawal from tamoxifen therapy.

Western medicine readily acknowledges that "the treatment of tamoxifen-induced hot flashes has been difficult." This is an important issue because hot flashes constitute the most common toxicity related to tamoxifen therapy. Unfortunately, women who experience tamoxifen-induced hot flashes really suffer. One study describes them as bothered not only during the day, but throughout the night. Many tamoxifen patients complained that hot flashes frequently woke them up and they found themselves drenched with perspiration, profuse enough to cause them to change their sheets and their nightclothes. Naturally, these tamoxifen users felt the after-effects of interrupted sleep during the day and also complained of tiredness.

In attempting to find solutions that can alleviate menopausal symptoms for women taking tamoxifen, a number of approaches have been tried. One was a transdermal patch, which unfortunately did not work well. In a 1994 issue of the *Journal of Oncology*, the study director stated that "Better means are needed to alleviate hot flashes among patients in whom estrogen therapy is contraindicated."

I believe that TCM, in general, and the *Wu Ming* Meridian Therapy taught in this book, in particular, can make a major contribution to menopause induced by drug therapies such as tamoxifen.

As we've seen, TCM understands menopausal symptoms as related to an imbalance in the body's overall Qi, and the dysfunction of the five major organ systems, mostly the liver. For many centuries, this diagnosis has been described in TCM medical texts. Today, in colleges and universities of TCM in the East as well as the West, hot flashes, vaginal discharge, and menstrual irregularities are readily identified as a Qi deficiency. This ancient medical system specifically relates these conditions to liver Qi stagnation and kidney Qi deficiency, as well as a disharmony between the way these two organs function and communicate with each other.

If you're suffering from tamoxifen-induced menopausal symptoms, all of the natural, self-healing treatments outlined in this book can help you a lot. In particular, *Wu Ming* Meridian Therapy with my Chinese herbal formulas can make a major contribution as adjuvant therapy for tamoxifen treatment. The result is that most women should be able to alleviate tamoxifen's side effects and continue hormone treatment.

To follow is a chart that lists the most common menopausal symptoms, their immediate causes, and their root causes. If you have any of these symptoms, study their root causes, then refer to Chapter 15 to see which organs or meridians can be helped with which foods and herbs. You can also fill out the questionnaire in the appendix and rate your symptoms. As you work with the information in this book, you can monitor your own healing progress. The TCM chart below clearly shows how the diverse discomforts of menopause can be traced back to their root causes—kidney Qi deficiency and liver Qi stagnation.

ROOT CAUSES OF MENOPAUSAL SYMPTOMS
ACCORDING TO TCM

MENOPAUSAL SYMPTOMS	IMMEDIATE CAUSE	ROOT CAUSE
Hot flashes/night sweats	Deficient yin Qi	Kidney/mother of liver; child of lung
Irritability/anger/ depression/nervousness	Poor function/disharmony of kidney, liver, lung	Liver/regulator of the flow of body's Qi
Anxiety/overworry	Poor liver function/stagnant liver Qi—whole body's Qi does not flow properly; Spleen/stomach partnership affected as well	Liver/regulates flow of whole body's Qi Liver: wood (liver) controls earth spleen)
Insomnia	Heart is too hot; deficient yin Qi and/or blood	Kidney: water (kidney) controls fire (heart)
Diarrhea, loose stool	Weak spleen (dampness)	Liver
Nausea, indigestion	Spleen/stomach	Liver
Bloating	Poor liver function— insufficient flow of Qi	Liver
Weight gain	Weak spleen—body cannot process food, holds onto fat and water	Liver
Joint pain	Liver governs tendon and ligaments	Liver
Muscle aches	Spleen—governs muscles	Liver
Vaginal dryness/loss of sex drive	Deficient kidney Qi	Kidney
Urinary infections	Deficient urinary bladder Qi	Kidney—yin/yang relationship with bladder
Skin problems	Lung—governs the skin	Kidney
Osteoporosis	Kidney—governs bones	Kidney
Heart problems/function problems	Heart too hot; deficient Qi, and/or blood	Kidney

TO SUMMARIZE:

- If you are experiencing symptoms such as hot flashes, night sweats, and vaginal dryness, and you're over forty, then most likely menopause has arrived.
- Other signs are a decrease in the frequency of periods, loss of sex drive, urinary infections, abnormal mood swings, digestive problems, shortness of breath, and heart palpitations.
- Hot flashes and night sweats are your body's signals that you have a kidney Qi deficiency.
- Liver Qi stagnation aggravates all menopausal symptoms.
- Hot flashes or sweats that occur during the day are usually due to a yang Qi deficiency; if they occur during the night, they are due to a yin Qi deficiency.
- Mood swings are usually caused by unbalanced liver function.
- The root cause of digestive problems is a disruption in the relationships between the liver, spleen, and kidney.
- Vaginal problems are caused by a kidney Qi deficiency and liver Qi stagnation.
- Reduced sexual desire has its root cause in deficient kidney Qi.
- Palpitations have their root cause in the disruption of the relationship between the kidney and the heart. Shortness of breath is due to a problem with the relationship between the kidney and lung.
- Menopause may occur naturally, or it can be caused by the removal of the uterus and ovaries, or it can develop as a result of drug treatments, such as tamoxifen.

The ancient wise man teaches us that if you can avoid the six environmental factors that cause health problems, if you can float in the mind of the Universe, if you can have less desire and attachment to earthly things, if you can strengthen your internal Qi, and if you can cradle your spirit within your heart, then where can disease come from and how can it enter?

Therefore, you should live with less desire and little expectation.

Then, you can live with a peaceful mind without panic. You can perform physical activity without depleting strength.

Your Qi can flow freely, and harmony and longevity can be yours.

NEI JING (475–221 B.C.)

CHAPTER 9

HOW TCM ADDRESSES THE THREE BIGGEST HEALTH PROBLEMS OF POSTMENOPAUSE
Heart Problems, Breast Cancer, Osteoporosis

*H*EART disease, breast cancer, and osteoporosis are the three major health problems that women fear as they age. TCM regards each, in turn, from the perspective of its root cause and which organ or organs have created the problem. TCM believes the first defense against these conditions is the creation of strong stomach Qi. Without a well-functioning stomach, you have no effective way to combat these diseases. As the *Nei Jing* says: "If you have stomach Qi, you have life. Without it, you are dead." In other words, stomach Qi is your lifeline to longevity. Let me show you why this is so.

When I first start working with patients, no matter what age, my first step is to strengthen their stomach's function, because almost always it's in poor condition. If I don't fix this problem first, then no matter how powerful an herbal formula I give them, no matter how brilliant an herbal concoction I can create, if their bodies can't process it very well, then we've lost the game. This is true of everything you put into your mouth—no matter what. If your stomach can't perform its assigned functions properly, you will get very little benefit from any foods, drugs, tonics, vitamins, minerals, supplements, nutraceuticals, energy boosters, or anything else for that matter that you ingest.

Why do Western people almost always have poor stomach function? From my experience with thousands of Western patients, I believe it's because the Western lifestyle is so stressful and Western eating habits are so unbalanced. Without an understanding of how the body works as a unified system, many people brush off this vital information. I'm sure you can relate to the following.

Look at what we do to ourselves almost every day. Our eating times are erratic. Even if you're hungry, you don't always get to eat on time. When you eat, you might overeat because you're so hungry. Or, you might work late, come home, eat a big meal late at night then go right to sleep. I can't tell you how bad this is for your stomach. And, you may repeat this pattern day after day, week after week, month after month.

Eating before bedtime can often cause sleep disturbances. TCM says, "If your stomach does not function very well, insomnia can be your nightly companion." This kind of insomnia can initiate a bad cycle. When you wake up, you're not hungry, so you skip breakfast in favor of getting something like a doughnut or bagel and coffee mid-morning. Or, you might need to eat something with a lot of sugar to satisfy your spleen's needs (remember its taste is sweet), then you go to work. The same busy and stressful day occurs again. The next thing you know, this has become your permanent unhealthy lifestyle.

Western lifestyles also create stomach function disorders because of the amount of food we eat and our choice of certain foods. There are so many restaurants and fast food places that advertise "all you can eat." And, many people do just that. This kind of overeating, especially if it becomes a habit, can cause serious havoc with your digestion system. No one really "needs" to eat a sixteen-ounce steak. No one really needs to eat platters and platters of fried shrimp! The Chinese have a saying, "You eat for the pleasure of your mouth and you eat as if it were for someone else's stomach."

Often Western diets are not varied enough either. They contain too much dairy food, too much sugar, too much alcohol, as well as too many cold foods and cold drinks. TCM understands that these things are active agents that, over time, can destroy the healthy workings of the stomach. If a stomach function disorder progresses, hypoglycemia or diabetes can result. Please be sure you test yourself with the TCM self-healing checklist on eating habits in Chapter 11. You might be very surprised at what you learn about foods and eating habits.

If you add the daily stresses that each of us undergoes, you also have an additional factor aggravating yet another organ: your liver. With this organ falling out of balance with the organ it's supposed to control, you can see how easy it is to begin to lose the battle to maintain the delicate balance of yin and yang energies that is essential to well-being. You may now experience stomach distention or bloating. You also may develop ulcers. For centuries, TCM has had tremendous success treating ulcers by reversing the "Liver Overcontrolling Stomach" condition. Once the stomach falls out of balance, you can almost guarantee that weight gain will follow, that you'll start to retain water in your body, to have loose stools, and you may even start to lose your hair.

If you go back and study the Five Element Theory Chart once more, you'll see that the stomach, which is the earth element, controls the kidney, which is the water element. When these organs are in balance, your body's all right. What happens when they become unbalanced? Think of an earthen dam. When the dam isn't strong enough to control the waters behind it, the waters will break through and flow everywhere. Treating the stomach lets us build up this dam and make it strong so that the waters behind are protected and controlled. This is the first step in treating the root cause of these three diseases that cause so much fear in women today. Prevention from as well as healing for heart disease, breast cancer, and osteoporosis depends on strong stomach Qi.

HEART DISEASE

We know that heart disease is the number one killer of women. We've seen that in TCM, the heart is the king of the organs, controlling the whole body's physical activity and Qi function. Because the heart is the king, it is very difficult to unseat and slow to suffer a physical problem in and of itself.

Whenever the heart does have a problem (unless it's related to a birth or genetic defect), TCM understands that it is always the result of a disrupted relationship with another organ. TCM regards the heart as the strongest organ. If it gets sick, TCM treats the pericardium, the heart's defender, instead of the heart itself. Or, it treats the heart through its related organs: the kidney that controls it, or the stomach, which is its child. Here again, we can see the elegance, flexibility, and ingenious ways that TCM theories open up many different paths for treating any one health problem.

From the Five Element Theory, we've learned that the heart controls the element of fire; it needs to be restrained and balanced by the water of the kidney. Although every organ needs the support of the kidney, this is especially true of the heart. As kidney Qi declines with age, it is less able to cool, quiet, and balance with the heart's Qi. If the kidney doesn't have enough power to control the heart, the fire of the heart burns out of control and can cause many problems.

If there are no physical defects in the heart or arteries, and no family history of heart disease—in other words, if heart problems are not physical, but functional—TCM understands that the true root cause is not to be found in the heart, but in the kidney. Symptoms of poor heart function often appear during or after menopause. They can include palpitations, other abnormal cardiac rhythms, insomnia, and high blood pressure. The catalyst for these conditions is a kidney Qi deficiency that leaves the proper function of the heart unsupported.

With many heart problems, strengthening the kidney is the main focus of TCM treatment. And this treatment, as always in TCM, is designed to be not only curative but preventive. If a woman can increase her kidney Qi during menopause, and learn how to take care of herself well, she will be much less likely to suffer from serious heart problems as she grows older.

Remember that we discussed that one of the heart's function

is mental activity. In my opinion, meditation is the best healing exercise. Meditation is a superior way to reduce excess mental activity and, believe it or not, repair yourself from the inside out. Meditation can complement all your self-healing activities during menopause. It is one of the true keys to longevity. On the physical and Qi levels, it can kill two birds with one stone: by meditating, you can conserve kidney Qi, which means this organ doesn't have to work so hard to protect your heart. In addition, your heart also doesn't have to work so hard to maintain its relationships with the other organs. When your heart function improves, your whole body functions better.

Meditation is something you can do anytime, anywhere, and under just about any condition. There is walking meditation, sitting meditation, standing meditation, and sleeping meditation. Meditation is the one thing you can practice for the rest of your life. It doesn't require any special machine; no special place; no special time; no special clothing. If you make regular meditation part of your life, I believe you will see tremendous health benefits.

When I teach meditation, one of the first things people often tell me is they don't have enough time to practice. I tell them there is both quality and quantity—you may not have hours on end to meditate, but I will let you in on a small secret. If you simply meditate a few minutes, even two minutes at a time, you can easily accumulate twenty minutes of meditation a day. How? When you're in your car in the morning, before you turn on the engine, sit quietly for a minute. That won't change your day. When you start your day, before you turn on your computer, before a major decision, before a big meeting, give yourself two small minutes (only 120 seconds!) to meditate. Before you go to bed or if you're in the bed, take two minutes before you go to sleep and before you get up. There are so many small spaces throughout your day that you can fill with only two minutes of meditation. Challenge yourself to find these special healing moments. You'll find that you'll have the ability to expand time. This way can also help you calm down and alter your current life's pattern so that you can save your Qi or healing energy. I recommend you go back to Chapter 6 and reread the section on the heart. It just might help save your life.

BREAST CANCER

Breast cancer is the most frequently diagnosed cancer for women in the United States. Most women are aware of the statistics. More than 180,000 new cases are diagnosed yearly. Annually, breast cancer claims more than 46,000 lives. After heart disease, breast cancer ranks as the number two killer of women. In this country, women have a one in eight lifetime risk of developing breast cancer.

The risk of developing breast cancer increases with age. The same conditions that are the source of menopausal symptoms are also at the root of breast cancer: kidney Qi deficiency and poor liver function. In the TCM view, the kidney controls a broad complex of functions including those that relate to the endocrine and immune systems. The liver controls the stomach, whose meridians—along with those of the liver—pass through the breasts. Unless you make a concerted effort to take care of yourself, the state of these organs will worsen with age. If you do not have breast cancer, the best way to prevent it is to focus on two things. Strengthen and harmonize your kidney Qi so that it can continue to produce adequate hormones even after menopause, and take steps to ensure that both your liver and stomach Qi flow smoothly and without blockage.

Breast cancer, like any disease, begins first as a Qi problem. When women complain of vague, intermittent discomforts that hardly ever show up on scientific tests, they are really speaking in the language of Qi. A good TCM doctor can understand and address these complaints immediately. What are some of them? You might experience breast tenderness intermittently. You might have headaches periodically, but not every day. When you rest they go away. You might take a few aspirin and things go back to normal. Western culture has conditioned us to believe these are insignificant events. They are not.

When a body is healthy it does not have physical, mental, or emotional problems. So, a TCM practitioner knows that these kinds of problems are the result of Qi imbalances. At this stage, it is relatively easy to fix these problems and prevent them from progressing to more serious conditions. The TCM patient learns to go to her doctor for small things because she has been educated to understand that prevention is the true cure. This might surprise many women who are afraid of not being "tough enough" or labeled a hypochondriac. A good TCM doctor wants to see you at the first sign of an imbalance or discomfort.

Any weakness or imbalance in the body's Qi will begin to cause function problems in the organs, although these symptoms may take some time to appear. If a functional disorder continues unchecked, physical evidence of it will eventually appear. A woman might begin to experience menstrual problems, PMS, breast tenderness, migraines, mood swings, and more. Not treated at the source, these physical symptoms can worsen and may lead to a precancerous condition. This is the time that masses or tumors can appear, or a woman may experience infertility or develop endometriosis.

Now, her problems have emerged in the physical world and they can indeed be seen and felt through scientific testing. If internal and external factors are right, then the physical problem can take a quantum leap and become cancer. Cancer's energy or Qi has overwhelmed the woman's own healing ability. If your Qi is strong enough and your organs function in harmony, this progression cannot occur. When your body functions this way, TCM says it is impossible for disease or illness to enter.

For those who want more information on breast cancer and TCM, I have written a comprehensive book on this subject called *Traditional Chinese Medicine: A Woman's Guide to Healing from Breast Cancer,* available from Avon Books. In it, I discuss how TCM had identified the root cause of breast cancer and ways to address it more than five hundred years ago. This is in contrast with the American Cancer Society's statement in its *Cancer Facts & Figures 1996:* "To date, knowledge about the risk factor has not translated into practical ways to prevent breast cancer."

Certain other factors also increase a woman's vulnerability to breast cancer: a family history of the disease, stomach problems, serious PMS, including breast distention and tenderness, and never having breast-fed a baby. If you're more at risk for cancer, you have to be more careful, and make more of an effort to take care of yourself. But I also want to emphasize that TCM believes even if you have a family history of breast cancer, it doesn't mean you will develop the disease yourself. You may be carrying the seed, but again if you can keep your Qi strong and your organs working together in harmony, you can keep cancer's seed under control with your own healing ability. You can keep it from developing. You can still live a good life and breast cancer will not kill you.

Breast cancer, and other cancers begin with Qi stagnation. Many women develop a Qi stagnation. From this stage, it is your lifestyle that determines whether or not this condition of Qi buildup will progress to a physical mass and whether the mass will turn cancerous. If you get breast cancer, TCM believes that, no matter what stage you are at in its progression, it is still possible to control cancer—to fight it and to win. You always have the potential to rebalance your Qi system from a state of disease to a state of health—or if not a state of health, at least a state wherein you and the condition can coexist peacefully.

At menopause, women have a difficult dilemma to face. They are afraid to begin HRT and they are afraid not to. If they begin, there is an increase in their risk of breast cancer, yet they are also told that HRT will protect them from heart disease and osteoporosis. According to the Center for Disease Control, women on HRT for 15 years have a risk factor that rises by 30%; their real risk rises an actual 3%. Suppose you're fifty years old and you will be on HRT for 15 more years, your risk of cancer has now risen to 13%. At sixty-five, however, which concern is more important, breast cancer or osteoporosis? When they are in their sixties, I think most women would say that breast cancer presents a much greater risk of dying than osteoporosis. Remember, with the proper support, Qi-fortifying practice, and lifestyle changes, your body can manufacture enough hormones naturally for the rest of your life.

I have a patient who was born with only one kidney, which developed cancer. His doctors gave him three months to live. My advice to him was simple: "Why don't you just try to enjoy yourself? Do something that you love." He went off to Florida and has been living there happily for three years now. When you're happy, your flow of Qi or life force is at its strongest and smoothest. Even if you have cancer, if you can stay positive and really let go, it's possible to defy the death sentence of doctors, and go on living for many years. This is not "happy talk," it is solidly grounded in the theories of a medical system that has been practiced continuously and successfully for more than five thousand years, right up until today! Remember the power to keep yourself alive comes from the spirit of your heart.

OSTEOPOROSIS

Osteoporosis affects one quarter of Caucasian American women. If a woman can strengthen herself and slow the decline of kidney Qi during and after her menopausal years, she may well be able to prevent bone problems such as osteoporosis in old age. Osteoporosis is a very frightening prospect. But if a woman turns to Western treatment with hormones to prevent it, she may not have the chance to live long enough for osteoporosis to be a problem. Why not go to the root cause instead? By strengthening the body's whole energy system you can not only avoid such problems, but live a life of less suffering and less stress.

According to the ancient Five Element Theory, each of the major organs governs a particular part of the body. Bones are the "tissue" of the kidney. Bones get their nourishment and the ability to promote the growth of new bone tissue from this organ. Thus, the health of the bones is directly connected to healthy kidney function.

Here are three major infant developments that demonstrate how kidney Qi and bones are related. They involve the teeth, the fontanels, and the knees. In a healthy baby, teeth, which TCM considers excess bone, grow quickly. The fontanels on the top of the baby's head will also close. And, at the proper time, the baby will also be able to stand up. If problems in any of these areas develop during early childhood, TCM will go straight to the root cause and treat the baby's kidney first. This practice has gone on for thousands of years and is still used successfully today.

Now, here's something I think you will find very interesting. Look at the other end of life. As we age, what happens? We lose our teeth. Then, we find that we're susceptible to weakness in the knees. And often, women in transition get headaches at the top of their head where branches of the kidney and liver meridians run. This problem relates to both organs. Today one of the most effective formulas in use for treating menopausal symptoms was developed in the twelfth century by the man considered to be the first Chinese pediatrician, Dr. Qian (A.D. 1032–1113).

Orthopedics is one of China's ancient specialties. For thousands of years, doctors of TCM developed protocols and classical herbal formulas to treat a wide variety of bone problems. In the case of a broken bone, for instance, TCM will always treat the kidney, trying to increase kidney Qi with herbs and foods such as bone soup. If the kidney can be strengthened, bones will heal much faster. One of the masters that I trained with could treat a broken bone overnight by prescribing an herbal formula to be taken internally and applying herbs externally. His skill was legendary in China. Many times, I witnessed this extraordinary healer treat people with broken bones in this amazing fashion. I was inspired by him and he helped fuel my interest in the traditional Chinese medical arts.

No matter what, because we are all under the natural law, sooner or later our bones tend to grow weaker with age and become much more susceptible to breakage. When kidney Qi declines, there is a definite loss of bone density, and these structures can become brittle. This is the cause of osteoporosis, and other degenerative bone diseases.

TCM's approach to treatment of osteoporosis looks at the

whole picture of how an individual takes care of herself. Its two treatment objectives are to focus on increasing kidney Qi first and then on strengthening the digestive system. As we age, our Qi income and expenditure tend to become unbalanced: we spend more Qi than we generate.

Again, you can see why it's very important to maximize the nutrition you get from the foods you eat. This means not only eating well, but improving the function of the digestive system. If your body cannot process food properly and extract the food's Qi, it doesn't matter what you eat. The same is true of supplements. Taking calcium for your bones is not going to help you very much if the organ responsible for processing it is working inefficiently. Your body will be too weak to absorb and utilize it. This applies to herbs as well, because you need strong digestion in order to extract their Qi. While some Western treatments offer some benefits, none go to the source and treat the root problem of the kidney.

The best way to treat osteoporosis is to address its root cause and understand the value of prevention. This means treating the liver and the kidney. I find that both my *Green Dragon* and *Imperial Qi* Formulas are very effective for all stages of menopause, even osteoporosis. If you want to avoid bone problems, I recommend that you make sure you keep your kidney Qi as strong as possible. You can start this very day. How do you do that? Eat for healing; incorporate as much seafood, including salmon, clams, oysters, lobsters, and shrimp; soy products, nuts, beans of all kinds, into your regular diet as possible. Find those minutes throughout the day when you can meditate as we discussed earlier.

Sooner or later, everyone develops some degree of bone deterioration. It is nature's way. We all wish our bones could stay as strong as they were when we were young. The reality is this isn't possible. What can we do? We can slow down the rate at which bone deterioration occurs. While there are exercises to increase muscle strength, and exercises for cardiovascular health, there are no bone exercises. But, there are classical herbs that can help strengthen kidney Qi and help the body function in harmony. If you have developed osteoporosis, you are now in need of some professional TCM help. At this time, you should try to find a skill-ful practitioner who understands how to rebalance your body's overall energy and strengthen your kidney Qi. Most likely, he or she will use acupuncture and herbs. The *Wu Ming* Meridian Therapy movements in Chapter 13 can also help strengthen the kidney, which is the engine that controls bone health. Be sure to pay particular attention to movement Number Eight. The longer you hold this posture, the more benefit you will gain.

If you're in your late forties or fifties and have developed os-teoporosis, and you have other physical problems such as diabetes, high blood pressure, high cholesterol, or you've been on lots of drugs, then your body is in crisis. It is struggling with the deep, fun-damental problem of kidney Qi deficiency. Additionally, all five major organ systems are out of balance and not functioning in har-mony. Naturally, this kind of severe condition takes much longer to fix. Coping with multiple problems obviously puts a tremendous strain on your whole system—body, mind, spirit, and emotions. The younger you are when you are diagnosed with osteoporosis, the harder you will have to work to heal yourself. You have over-drawn your Inborn Qi to such an extent that you are now experi-encing an older person's condition. You've accelerated your own aging process. This requires an all-out effort to change your lifestyle, to readjust the pace of your everyday life, to change your eating habits, and to transform negative thinking and emotional re-actions.

The wise man shows us the way to longevity.

When the seasons change, we should mirror these changes.

Challenging nature is futile.

Keeping a peaceful mind and living a simple life without undue desire allows the energy of the Universe to flow through you.

If your body, mind, and spirit become one, where is the space for illness?

NEI JING (475–221 B.C.)

CHAPTER 10

TCM:
Treating the Source, Not
the Symptoms of Menopause

*R*ACHEL is a fifty-seven-year-old schoolteacher who had had chronic fatigue syndrome for six years. When she first came to see me she was also experiencing hot flashes, vaginal dryness, lack of sexual interest, frequent urination at night, insomnia, and had swollen ankles. By examining her, I found that she had a severe kidney Qi deficiency. I gave her acupuncture as well as herbs in the form of capsules. She came to see me once a week, every week for five weeks.

By the fourth visit, she began to sleep well. She got up to urinate only twice a night rather than five times. Her hot flashes went away; swelling in her ankles went down, and her fatigue and vaginal dryness improved. After five more treatments, her constipation improved about 80 percent; the vaginal dryness and fatigue completely healed. Rachel returns twice a year for her energy "tune-up" or "acupuncture acu-torture," as many of my patients like to call it. Now she says, "I feel ten years younger. I really feel better than I did when I thought I had a lot of energy years ago!"

Let's look at menopause the way TCM sees it. First, it regards the presenting symptom (Rachel's hot flashes and other symptoms, for example) as a signal from the body of a deeper situation that is affecting either an organ or a meridian (or both) that must be addressed. However, virtually all women who come to me with menopausal symptoms suffer from the same things: a deficiency of kidney Qi and/or stagnation of liver Qi. But I never leave anything to chance, because there might be other problems going on as well. Therefore I see Rachel's symptoms as being unique to her own special energy pattern. In other words, Rachel's hot flashes and constipation are not the same as yours or your girlfriend's, or your mother's, or your colleague's, even if you all share the same characteristics. Why? Quite simply because her symptoms are hers alone and not anyone else's. Likewise your symptoms are unique.

As we've seen, rather than naming the condition, TCM diagnoses it in terms of either an energy or Qi function disorder or a Qi imbalance, as these states relate to the particular organ(s) or meridian(s) that are distressed. One more example that might help you understand how TCM views health conditions relates to migraine headaches. Once again, your migraine headache is not the same as your girlfriend's, or your mother's, or your colleague's, even if they share all the same characteristics. Why? The answer is the same; you are not they and they are not you.

Unless there is a tumor, nerve damage, or blood clots, TCM considers headaches the result of Qi stagnation. If you have had all kinds of tests like x-rays, CT scans, MRIs, etc., to identify the cause of your headache, and the results are normal, your headache is the result of Qi or energy stagnation. According to TCM theories, wherever you have pain you have a Qi blockage.

In the case of headaches, TCM identifies six major meridians (all yang Qi meridians rise up) that either start or end in the head. A Qi blockage in any one meridian or a combination of meridians can cause your migraine. Here's an analogy that might help you understand this concept better. Think about a city with six major highways; if even one of them is blocked, there will be a traffic jam; if more than one highway becomes blocked, in any combination with the other five roads, there will also be a big problem. Simple math tells us then that there are 720 (6 x 5 x 4 x 3 x 2 x 1 = 720) different combinations that have the potential to cause a traffic jam.

It's exactly the same with headaches. TCM recognizes that Qi blockages can result from seven hundred twenty different possibilities. So, it's unlikely that you'll find two headaches that are exactly alike. When a man has a migraine headache at the side of his head, suppose he uses the best-selling analgesic. When his wife has a side headache at the same spot during her menstrual cycle, she may take the same painkiller and find no relief. Why? Her headache is different from his. The root cause of their headaches is different. Looking at it this way, you can gain a better insight into why some over-the-counter medication works for some people and not for others.

From the TCM standpoint, everything about you is unique. Consequently, TCM focuses its attention on your individual problem-producing dynamics. By treating you as an individual, TCM can treat your migraine effectively. How? It can get to the root cause of it. If you have a health problem, your body is out of balance and offers the ideal environment within which unbalanced Qi can comfortably reside. Without the right kind of help to rebalance your organ system, this condition is unlikely to resolve itself on its own. The real healer helps create the opportunity for the patient to change her energy field, reawaken her healing ability, and reconnect to her state of internal harmony. Reaching this means reaching the root cause of the problem. If you can do this, then your condition, in this case menopausal symptoms, can be healed. Here are the main treatment principles of TCM.

TCM TREATMENT PRINCIPLES

- Treat the root cause.
- Strengthen the body's immune system.
- Harmonize the function of the body's organs.
- Adapt treatment to the specific needs of the individual: "who you are" (body type, genetics), "where you are" (geographical location); "how you are" (physical and emotional condition and lifestyle); and "when you are" (age, time of day and season, time of symptom).

The various treatments discussed in this chapter must be applied using the above principles. How does TCM approach treatment? The TCM practitioner is trained to understand that effective treatment always depends on: who you are; where you are; how you are; and when you are. In other words, your current condition and genetic blueprint, your physical location, current physical condition and habits, time (your age, time of day, or season), are all specific factors that determine the course (and the outcome) of your treatment. The more knowledgeable a TCM practitioner is the more data he searches for to give him more clues to your problem. The less knowledgeable practitioner only treats the symptoms.

A good TCM doctor bases the selection of treatments on two objectives: to address the root cause and to prevent the problem from going deeper and affecting other organs.

The initial step in this process is to determine whether the symptoms indicate an emergency or whether they represent some sort of chronic condition. TCM treatments include herbal therapy, acupuncture, Chinese medical massage, known as *Tuina* or acupressure, Qigong, the skillful prescription of healing foods, and the application of ancient psychology. Above all, TCM recognizes the body's capacity to heal itself and works at nurturing this ability. The true specialty of TCM is prevention.

I'm often asked if certain conditions respond better to TCM than to Western medicine. There are many that do. TCM is good for strengthening the immune system and for treating chronic conditions like systemic lupus erythematosus (SLE), chronic stomachaches or headaches, chronic fatigue syndrome, allergies, asthma, skin problems, and hypoglycemia, to name a few. These kinds of internal problems take time and patience to heal and to gain maximum results, but the exciting part is that the root cause is being addressed so that the condition can be eliminated or dramatically altered. For conditions like tennis elbow, sprains, stiff necks, and muscle pulls, TCM is often faster and more effective than Western treatment, especially since there are no side effects.

A good many of the Western women who come to see me are pretty much at the end of their ropes. As you've seen from the stories in this book, a number of them have suffered for many years and tried many things to rid themselves of their health problems. Some have spent small fortunes and gone for longer than a decade in search of relief. Often I see a patient who has undergone a battery of Western medical tests and who has been told that she is "fine." The patient, however, is acutely aware that she is not fine (nor is she crazy—as some of my patients have been told). Often, dramatic changes can occur in relatively brief treatment periods if we communicate well and work together productively. I think some of the case histories outlined here give you a good idea of why and how this can happen. These changes are not the result of "quick fixes." Routinely, they are permanent reversals of conditions that have been addressed by finally treating the source and not the symptoms.

My first-time patients are often unaware of what to expect from a visit to a TCM doctor. In my practice, my first order of business is to explain that I am a classically trained doctor of TCM. I am not a Western medical doctor with some TCM training. My classical training lies rooted in the tradition of the best ancient doctors. These individuals were, above all, expected to be Qigong or energy masters and deeply versed in the understanding of Qi, because Qi is the foundation of all traditional Chinese medicine. They were also expected to be expert martial artists, because the martial arts are intended for healing first and self-defense second.

Another skill required of them was the ability to make up ancient herbal formulas in the TCM apothecary and, when needed, adapt them to the specific needs of each patient. They were also taught how to apply TCM's fundamental principles and theories, including the Five Element Theory, Ying and Yang, Meridian and Organ, and Qi and Blood to their patients' conditions. Without this kind of deep training and experience with Qi, it is still possible to practice the techniques of TCM, but not its true spirit and power. Many of these ancient doctors were also passed information from their masters.

One of my goals is to educate my patients and help them understand that Qi is the real secret behind TCM. No matter which technique is used, be it herbs, or foods, or acupressure, or acupuncture, the real secret behind these treatments is always Qi. The challenge is for the energy practitioner to spark the patient's own Qi to respond. You can compare this with a car that needs a jump start because its battery has died. If the battery is in good shape, a good charge will make it work again.

My own master, Professor Xi-hua Xu of Yunnan, China, continually reminds me that a good healer must first begin by creating an energy bond between the doctor and the patient. Without this Qi connection, no matter how good a doctor, the treatment process can only take place at the symptom level. But, with a strong Qi connection or bond, the healer and patient can actually amplify their energy field exponentially, to help the individual's own healing power to overcome disease or illness.

Because TCM views the treatment process as a partnership, it is vital that both partners get to know each other. It is the whole person, not the disease, that requires attention—her body, mind, and spirit—if good results are to be gained. Therefore, psychological issues always bear on the ultimate success of the treatment. Spending time with the patient is an essential part of TCM treatment. You can begin to appreciate the difference between the TCM and Western approaches to treatment of illness and disease and healing.

Because modern society causes so many stress-related conditions and today's lifestyles are so complicated, the skilled TCM practitioner spends a lot of time sorting out with the patient just how they got sick or out of balance in the first place. This is the first step in helping the patient identify the root cause of her condition. Without this step, the healing process will be slow and cannot produce a dramatic change. Why? Because only the practitioner is doing the job. The patient must learn how to help herself so she can recognize and avoid the situations and lifestyle habits that made her ill in the first place.

As we've seen, TCM believes emotions and organs are inextricably linked, so it is essential to help the patient realize that her unbalanced emotional reactions to situations may, at the deepest level, be the root cause of her physical problems. This is not the same as saying that a patient's problem is "all in her head." Sometimes this concept is misunderstood because in the West there is no organized framework for comprehending how the energy of excess emotions can affect and even damage their corresponding organs. When you begin to understand the energetic power the five major emotions have on the *physical* condition of their related organs, disease and illness can be seen from a much deeper perspective.

We learn from meditation that: "Your heart can create heaven or hell." To put it into more modern terms: "It's not what happens to you, but how you take it." For TCM, emotional, psychological, and spiritual factors are crucial parts of the puzzle; without this mutual understanding of the healer and the patient and the context of the theories of Qi and Blood, Yin and Yang, and Five Element, treatment is incomplete.

It is helpful to a new patient to describe what she can expect in her upcoming appointment. I tell her the TCM exam is made up of four diagnostic methods: looking (facial color, shape, eye and tongue color, emotional state); smelling and hearing (body and mouth odor, noise from the chest and nose); asking (talking about the patient's problem—especially probing for clues that relate to frequency, time of day, degree, type), and touch (including pulse diagnosis). I try to educate her about the organs and their associated emotions so that she begins to see how emotional problems can cause physical ones.

It is essential for me as a TCM practitioner to understand how my patient "feels" and what kind of emotional or spiritual issues are affecting her life. I am constantly looking for clues to help her resolve her health issues from her physical form, her internal health condition, and from the state of her soul or spirit. Of these three factors, the state of her spirit is, by far, the most important one. TCM believes that if you have spirit, you have life; if the spirit is gone, there is nothing either one of us can do. If a patient has breast cancer, it is important to spend quality time with her, especially to encourage her spirit to continue its fight.

By treating you as an individual, TCM can treat your menopausal symptoms effectively, and above all, find the key to help your body, mind, and soul heal themselves. I have written this book to help women understand how to take the initiative to heal themselves. I want all women approaching menopause to know that TCM can offer a healthier alternative to hormone replacement therapy. Working with so many Western women made me realize that any book I wrote would need a comprehensive, yet clear explanation of the TCM process. In this chapter, I'd like to do just that. Let's take the time to explore in detail what to expect from a visit to a TCM practitioner.

THE FIRST VISIT TO A TCM DOCTOR

When new patients make an appointment, I ask them to fill out our TCM Personal Self-Healing Evaluation Form to help me understand the condition of their major organs, as well as their emotional state. In my practice, we use the same form that's included in the Appendix of this book. It specifically relates to menopausal problems and can help you evaluate your current condition. I suggest you make several copies of it. This way you can work with the information in this book, week by week, and chart your progress toward good health.

Looking

There are three things I "look" at: the first is spirit, the second is Qi, the third is the physical form and how it's functioning. Spirit is by far the most important factor I consider. I look first at your "spirit," asking myself "What is the state of this person's spirit?" I look at your eyes (which, as you know, is the window to the heart or spirit soul). I learn a great deal about your spirit from your eyes. I look at the spirit behind every physical aspect of you.

I then look at the shape of your body, the posture of your body—how you sit, how you stand, how you move, the emotions that play over your face as you talk with me. I also look at your tongue, both its shape and its color; your face, both its shape and its color, and the shape of your head. Your face might have different hues surrounding it: red, white, green, yellow, black. According to the Five Element Theory, each color is related to the Qi of one of your organs. Your physical face may not actually show these colors, but the aura you give off, which is related to your Qi, is evident to a trained TCM practitioner.

Your tongue's appearance is particularly critical in diagnosing the internal state of your organs. Even before you experience any symptoms, a problem will always show up on your tongue. A healthy tongue is pale red in color, moist with a thin white coating, and will fit easily in your mouth. If you have a bright red tongue and a dry mouth, especially at night, I would say that you have a yin Qi deficiency. If you have a pale tongue, it would reveal a yang Qi deficiency. A fat tongue with teethlike marks on the sides indicates an overall Qi deficiency. This is often seen with people who are undergoing chemotherapy or radiation. A tongue with a thick white coating tells me that your stomach or spleen has a great deal of internal dampness, indicating that you probably eat or drink too many cold things. If your tongue has a yellow coating and you have bad breath and constipation, I would say that your stomach suffers from too much heat. In TCM practice, the tongue is a valuable indicator of health problems.

As my patient describes her problems, I engage her in conversation and try to get her to talk freely. When this happens, I am able to observe her true spirit behind the physical form, and what emotional state she is in. Sometimes we may be chatting about weather or about nothing. At these moments, the TCM practitioner must pay close attention to the patient. At this time, I can see in my own patient that behind her polite conversation she wants to cry, but she is in such control and her emotions are so bottled up that she can't let go. If you are a good enough practitioner, you can catch these moments and gain insight into where the deeper problems of emotions lie. Many patients tell me sincerely that they are not angry or holding on to any angry feelings.

And, they truly mean this. Yet, when we discuss an incident in their lives, they will often exhibit signs of anger without being conscious of them. Their eyes will flash; their breathing will change; their voice will have a different tone. This deep-seated emotion has the ability to unbalance their liver function. I also ask my patients to walk a bit so that I can observe their balance and how strong their Qi is.

Smelling and Hearing

Another part of an evaluation includes using the senses of smelling and hearing to see if you have any body or mouth odor or whether you have noise coming from your chest and nose. It is important to hear the patient's voice. At this point, I ask her to talk so I can hear her voice, checking if it is high or low, strong or weak. I am very interested in where her voice is pitched so that I can tell how deep her Qi is and whether her voice comes from the soul. While hearing is a key tool, in my opinion, listening is one of the highest healing activities of the twentieth century. While ancient doctors possessed the skill of looking at patients without having them talk, today it is essential to help patients speak from their heart. Listening is an aspect of building a trusting relationship with my own patients. I find that most Western women have no place to go where they can talk from their heart to someone who wants to help them and who will actually listen to them. In building this trusting relationship, I can also give my patients a great deal of hope. When hope exists, people are willing to do a lot of things to help themselves heal.

Asking

This is the part of the examination when the TCM practitioner asks directly about your problems, and you ask your questions. In this area, I am very focused and ask very specific questions, because I am probing for clues that relate to the type of problem(s) you have, its frequency and degree, and time of day it occurs. I also want to know about your sleeping habits, your diet, and even when, where, and why you perspire. I might ask, "How well do you sleep at night?" "Do you wake up at a specific hour during the night?" or "What is your appetite like, and what are your favorite foods?" I also might ask you, "Where do you think this problem comes from?" "When did it start?" No matter how unusual the answer, I am always vitally interested in the patient's perspective on her own health condition. Intuitively, a lot of women can relate their problems to an emotional trigger or root cause, but often they've been talked out of this insight, or someone might say to them "That's ridiculous. Breast cancer, or pneumonia, or whatever . . . doesn't start that way. It's all in your mind!" Each one of my questions has a purpose. My master always tells me that a good doctor must ask the right questions at the right time to find out simple, yet vital, information.

Touching

Generally speaking, touching can be divided into the pulse diagnosis and the physical touch diagnosis. The first one helps the TCM doctor understand the internal energy condition of the organs. The second one helps the TCM doctor understand the condition of the body, for example, if you are injured, well-trained TCM doctors can distinguish by touch whether you have a fracture, a break, or a tendon problem. They can do this without relying on X rays, CT scans, or MRIs. Some special acupoints can be touched to determine if a specific organ has a Qi disorder. Some points can indicate to the TCM doctor whether or not cancer is present.

The pulse diagnosis speaks volumes to the TCM practitioner. Understanding the intricate vocabulary of the pulse diagnosis is a lifelong learning process. With a pulse diagnosis, a TCM practitioner is not just feeling the beating of a person's heart. Pulse diagnosis is a very ancient, highly sophisticated, and complex tool. During the exam, 24 different qualities of energy vibration—are checked with three fingers delicately pressing and releasing pressure along the radial artery. Each pulse is related to the Qi or life force of one of your organs.

	Left Wrist		Right Wrist
Heart	Small Intestine	Lung	Large Intestine
Liver	Gallbladder	Spleen	Stomach
Kidney	Bladder	Pericardium	Triple Warmer

The feel of the pulses enables a TCM doctor to understand the condition of your Qi, blood, the yin and yang Qi of the individual organs, Qi deficiencies or excesses, and your overall balance. Altogether, twenty-four qualities can be felt on each pulse, among them are frequency, speed, power, and feeling. Sometimes my patients are amazed that I can tell them the sex of their baby even though the fetus is only five-weeks-old. I like to let them know that there are many well-trained TCM doctors whose pulse diagnosis skills have the sensitivity to do this.

One of my patients, Carolyn who was sixty-one, came to see me because she was constipated and had been experiencing nightmares and insomnia. She also told me that her urine was very yellow and that she often had a very dry mouth. When I took her pulse, I "saw" that her heart pulse was very fast, which meant that her heart was experiencing a condition of "fire," or extreme heat. Given Carolyn's other symptoms and her age, I felt that the true source of her excess heat was not really her heart, but the result of a kidney Qi deficiency. So I treated both her kidney and heart with good success for both of us.

CHOOSING A DOCTOR OF TCM

It is not surprising that the use of alternative (I like to think of it as complementary) medicine, as it is called, is growing rapidly in the West. A 1998 study in the *Journal of the American Medical Association* states that alternative therapies are being used by four out of every ten Americans. The study also says that consumers spent $27 billion dollars on remedies ranging from herbal pills to acupuncture. It's interesting to note that most of these dollars are coming out of the consumer's own pocket. With so many people searching for answers to their health needs, it is important to know how to select knowledgeable, quality care. This is also very important when choosing a practitioner of TCM.

When a patient moves, I am often asked how to find a good TCM doctor. The truth is, it isn't easy. It is not like selecting a Western physician. When choosing a TCM practitioner, I tell my patients to trust their intuition. If the treatment isn't working within a short time, I tell her that she must talk things over with her TCM doctor to uncover why. If she does not feel that she can establish a trusting working partnership, if she does not observe the doctor's ability to skillfully apply the TCM principles and does not seem interested in identifying the root causes of her problem, then I advise her to find another doctor. Otherwise, I tell her "You are being treated in the Western way—substituting acupuncture needles for drugs, and substituting technique for theory. Your symptoms may be receiving treatment, and you might even be experiencing a certain degree of relief. However, the true source of your condition is still being ignored." It is also my responsibility to point out a very real danger in this situation. If the practitioner does not have a deep understanding of TCM principles and theories, he or she can do more harm to the patient than a Western doctor. Why? It's because they are dealing with the body's natural healing Qi. If the practitioner misdirects it, then he or she can cause more internal problems than when the patient started.

There are several ways you can identify whether or not a TCM practitioner has the kind of training and insight that can help you. For your own education, take the time to read over the main principles and theories of TCM in Chapters 3, 4, and 5. These have remained unchanged for many thousands of years. Also review the Five Element Theory so you can become familiar with the relationships among the five major organ pairs and the internal and external factors that influence their healthy function and balance. Try to see where your physical discomfort fits. What organs might it be related to? Which emotions may be playing a role in your problem? If you are healthy, you can apply all this knowledge to keep you well and prevent health issues, menopausal symptoms or conditions, from getting out of control.

Now when you select a practitioner of TCM you have some common ground. When you meet, does he or she use the classical four-stage diagnosis methodology outlined above? Second, does he or she take the time to create that indispensable energy bond with you, or do you get a ten-minute work-up and then get sent to a room for acupuncture treatment? (Remember it's the energy relationship that heals, the energy vehicle of the needles or herbs are of secondary importance.) Does he or she help you realize there are daily lifestyle choices that you must take responsibility for changing in order to heal? If you have no benefit after a few visits, does he or she sit with you to redesign treatment to get at the problem another way? Remember the dynamics of generation and control in the Five Element Theory offer the skilled TCM practitioner many paths for dealing with the same problem.

When you discuss your symptoms, can he or she work with you to identify factors that are causing them? For example, does your practitioner understand that your breast tenderness, PMS, and menstrual cramps are all related to a stressed lifestyle and a liver function disorder? Does he or she understand that your migraine headache that occurs each morning at 8:00 A.M. means that your stomach Qi is not functioning properly? When searching for a TCM doctor (or acupuncturist, or herbalist), I believe your best choice is one who understands and practices TCM in accordance with its ancient principles and theories. I also believe that one who practices Qigong and deeply believes in the power and principals of Qi can benefit you the most.

TCM TREATMENTS

As we've seen, the TCM practitioner's role is simple and complex at the same time. His or her job is to balance the opposing, yet complementary, yin and yang energies within the patient and strengthen her own healing ability so she can heal herself. TCM practitioners have a variety of vehicles to use for this purpose. They are: foods for healing, herbal therapy, acupuncture, acupressure, moxibustion (the application of heated herbs to a particular acupoint or meridian), Qigong, the ancient self-healing energy practice, and Chinese psychology. Now let's take a deeper look at each of these.

Food

Since ancient times, TCM has used food both to prevent and treat disease. The healing power of most medicines—even herbs—has the potential to harm. Only food has no poison. If you know how to choose foods based on their healing Qi, you can eat not just for survival, but for health. Food is our main source of postnatal Qi. The goal of eating for healing is to maximize the amount of Qi you get from food, and minimize the Qi it takes to digest it. Remember that you want to draw as much as possible on your checking account of Qi produced by the stomach, and as little as possible on your savings account of kidney Qi.

TCM has a long history of prescribing food as medicine. Ancient doctors understood, from an energy perspective, which foods could heal which organs. This information has been passed down and been in use for thousands of years. In Chapter 15, I have compiled a broad list of healing foods and classical herbs for women going through perimenopause and menopause, as well as how to use them. These are accompanied by healing recipes using these ingredients, which can help you a lot. They are useful whether you want to prevent or relieve uncomfortable symptoms. You now have the knowledge to apply this information in conjunction with your understanding of various symptoms. This can help heal certain early stage conditions so that they do not progress to bigger health problems. Start now. Begin today to work with these foods, you will be surprised at their ability to relieve menopausal symptoms and discomforts. To the best of my knowledge, this comprehensive healing resource has never been organized for Western audiences like this before.

Foods are natural elements and, when used properly, produce

virtually no side effects. Eating good quality foods everyday is something you can do to help yourself. TCM has a unique understanding of foods as medicine that goes beyond the physical properties of nutrition, calories, or vitamins. Long, long ago, TCM had mapped out the healing energies and essences of specific foods and the organs they go to. Do you remember how food becomes Qi or the power and intelligence to run the complex functions of your body? First the food comes into the body and turns into essence via the work of the spleen/stomach partnership; this nutritive essence is sent up to the lung where it receives its instructions about where to go. The lung, in turn, is so intelligent that it knows that each food is coded with its own essence and understands which organs it should be sent to.

What happens when you make a delicious soup with black beans, sweet potatoes, scallions, ginger, and cinnamon? After the stomach digests your food, the spleen will send the nutritive essence of each food to the lung. Then, the lung will transform these essences into Qi and distribute it to specific organs. The Qi of the black beans and cinnamon will go immediately to your kidney; the Qi or essence of the sweet potato and ginger will enter your stomach and spleen; the scallion's Qi will go directly to your liver. Each of these foods will help strengthen the organ to which they relate. This Qi blueprint is even more important than the foods' physical properties.

Today, there is a lot of ongoing research in the West as scientists attempt to prove conclusively that certain foods, like broccoli, carrots, kale, etc., can help prevent or treat certain conditions, such as breast cancer. Until science can go beyond the physical properties of food and apply the concept of Qi, how these foods benefit breast cancer patients might remain a mystery. TCM has known for centuries that certain foods can help heal the root cause of breast cancer. They have used these foods to break up Qi stagnation in the six meridians that run through the breast area. I have written about a wide variety of these food and healing herbs in my first book, *Traditional Chinese Medicine: A Woman's Guide to Healing from Breast Cancer*. Well-trained TCM doctors know how to create various food recipes for healing purposes. One of the most vital steps in the Seven-Point Guide to Self-Healing for Menopause is understanding how to eat for healing. Be sure and read Chapter 15 and use this information to restructure your eating habits so that you can address certain menopausal symptoms naturally.

The most important principle of healthy eating is to eat in a way that supports the function of the digestive system. You need to manage your spleen/stomach partnership very well, and to understand what these organs need to function harmoniously. Both of them like warmth; cold foods damage them. By "cold" I mean not only foods that are actually cold, such as ice cream and iced drinks, but foods that are cold by nature. Salads and raw vegetables are two good examples of cold foods. Some diets encourage eating lots of raw foods, because of the concern with losing nutrients in cooking. I would like you to understand that it's not a bad thing to eat raw vegetables once in a while, but your stomach has to spend a lot of its Qi to digest uncooked foods. From the TCM perspective, you end up losing more than you gain. The same is true of cold foods—the stomach has to spend too much Qi to warm them up, and then digest them.

At my workshops, I get a big reaction when I pass this ancient TCM knowledge on. Most Western people are a bit stunned by it. All their lives, in virtually every media outlet, in virtually every diet they've gone on, they've been told how important it is to eat large quantities of raw vegetables. I would like women dealing with menopausal symptoms to understand that to heal these conditions naturally, you must save every bit of Qi, or life force, you can and apply it to your healing process. It takes a good deal of Qi to heal health issues. Here is one easy opportunity once you understand how it works. If you love raw vegetables, learn to parboil them even for a few minutes before eating to help yourself conserve healing Qi, then study the foods in Chapter 15 and learn which ones carry warmth and which ones don't.

Another important principle of healthy eating is moderation. We're constantly being admonished either to eat or not to eat certain foods. But I believe you can eat just about anything in moderation. Whether or not you consume specific foods or substances—such as caffeine, alcohol, or foods high in cholesterol—is too small a focus. It's the big picture of adhering to the principles of healthy eating that counts. Many of us tend to eat a small number of favorite foods to excess.

I spend quite a bit of time with my patients discussing their eating habits. Here are some of my key recommendations. Try to keep your diet diverse and balanced. Don't eat too much food at one time. Eat until you're about 75 percent full. This leaves room for the normal digestive function to take place. If you overeat, you overspend your Qi to process the excess food. Eat a moderate amount of food at regular mealtimes. Don't eat a heavy meal before you go to bed. If this is one of your habits, you are on the way to major digestive problems, if you're not already suffering from insomnia.

If you watch your diet, eat a variety of healthy foods, and don't eat a lot of junk food, then don't focus on a cup of coffee, or a package of artificial sweetener, or worry about drinking low-fat milk. Incidentally, here's another area where I seem to disconcert my Western audiences. I recommend drinking real milk, not the low-fat kind. I usually make a joke and say "The cow doesn't give low-fat milk, or 2-percent milk. How did the milk get that way?" If you do the research, I think you'll learn that natural products are just better for you. Learn to eat them in moderation. For example, I like half-and-half in my coffee; I never worry about this because it's just one small thing. It is more important for me (and for you) to pay attention to your lifestyle, and the daily habits you have. When I talk with my patients, we sometimes laugh about some of our first conversations where they try to convince me (and themselves) that they are serious about getting well. They mention their artificial sweeteners, low-fat milk, reduced fat cookies, fifty-calorie breads, and in the next breath talk about hoping to quit smoking, cutting down on their fifty-hour workweek, and going to bed before 1:00 A.M. The intelligent and determined patients finally "get it" that they must focus on the big things, in other words, their whole lifestyle. They must create healthy ways to keep their emotions in balance, if they really want major healing benefits. This is especially true for women going through menopause. Don't fool yourself; focus on the real things that can help you make a quantum leap in health.

Try to listen to your body and tune in to what it's telling you it wants or doesn't want to eat. Don't automatically follow the cravings of your mind. Sometimes it's hard to tell the difference— "is it my mind that wants this, or my body?" But over time, especially as your Qigong practice progresses, you can develop a sensitivity to what is going on with your body's Qi.

Some women, particularly during their menstrual cycle have the experience of craving sugar or salt. At this time, your body is actually telling you that it's out of balance and needs this substance. For example, if your body yearns for sugar, be aware that this has to do with the poor function of your spleen (the organ corresponding with the sweet taste). If you have this kind of craving, you should eat what your body wants. Eating foods with some sugar or salt at this time can help you. You also need to support the function of your organs with foods that support their Qi. In the case of the spleen, some of these foods are sweet potatoes and yams, beans, corn, chestnuts, and lotus seeds. Incorporating them into your diet can eventually help you reduce your sugar craving. Eating seafood of all kinds, especially shrimp, lobster, clams, and oysters can also help reduce salt cravings.

TCM believes that it is better to get your Qi from food than from an additive to your diet. As far as vitamin and mineral supplements are concerned, if you're healthy and eat well, in my opinion, it's not necessary to take them. If the function of your digestive system is poor, it doesn't matter what you eat—according to TCM, a weak stomach does not have the power or strength to extract maximum Qi from the food, or supplements you put in it. If the function of your digestive system is good, and you eat nutritious food, why do you need supplements? Though you may gain some benefit from some supplements, no amount of these substances will compensate for or improve poor digestive function, nor should they be used as a replacement for nutritious food.

When I hold workshops on our Dragon's Way® weight loss program, people tell me that they've heard that the soil in America has been depleted of vitamins and minerals so that the food we eat in this country isn't nearly as nutritious as it should be. They tell me that this is a valid reason for taking lots of supplements. My response sometimes surprises them. I tell them that the soil in America has been cultivated intensively for less than three hundred years. Look at some of the other countries around the world. What about England's soil? What about Europe's? Or China's? Farmers in these places have cultivated their land for far longer than farmers in America. By rights, these people should also need tremendous amounts of supplements to remain well. But, this isn't really the case. Remember that nature has its own law and nature has its own capacity to heal itself. Even though we don't protect nature, it has its own power to readjust and recalibrate itself, so that it doesn't lose its healthy properties. Don't let this kind of worry influence you to purchase large quantities of vitamins, minerals, supplements, or the latest herbal ingredient. Trust your intuition and eat a variety of good quality foods on a regular basis.

TCM Herbs

Today many consumers try to help themselves when they're sick. This is especially true if they have a chronic condition that Western medicine cannot cure. Another group of consumers have the good intention of wanting to prevent disease or illness. Both groups frequently turn to natural food supplements, vitamins, tonics, herbal compounds, etc. You name the problem, whether it is osteoporosis, heart disease, brain function improvement, or sexual power, there is something on the market you can take that supposedly helps. I always tell my patients to think about this concept carefully: "You have a symptom; you take a pill for it." In the case of single herbs or herbal formulas, the only difference is that they are replacing chemical substances with natural compounds. They are still not treating the root cause.

Too often, I see patients ingesting large quantities of these pills, vitamins, minerals, and tonics. I ask them how they know if these things will help them? How do they know if they won't harm them? Most laboratories haven't tested this kind of real life usage (or abuse, in some cases), nor have they tested their products in these vast combinations. I also tell my patients to think twice before ingesting large quantities of these substances because they all must pass through the stomach, the liver, or the kidney.

A vast apothecary of herbs has been available to TCM practitioners for healing purposes for thousands of years. The goal of classical TCM herbal formulas is to treat the root cause and stimulate the organs to heal themselves. In the East, the concept of "herb" has a broader meaning than in the West. An herb can mean any natural material used in a formula. Ancient TCM doctors were skilled at using all kinds of things for healing. Stones, bones, dirt, glass, wood, bark, leaves, roots, petals, stems, and just about every conceivable animal body part could be included in an herbal recipe.

Classical TCM herbal remedies are based on a particular combination of selected herbs; the result is a unique medicine stronger than the sum of its parts. One way to understand this concept is to look at the TCM herbal ingredient as a football player—not a tennis player. In a TCM formulation, the team is what counts. Every herb has a specific job: some herbs are used to directly impact a given condition; some are used to help tune up certain organs; some help strengthen an organ's Qi or power; some are used to flush out toxic material; others block the disease or illness from becoming worse—anticipating its next move—and some herbs help create an inhospitable internal environment where the disease or toxic invader is no longer comfortable.

This last technique is very interesting. I'll give you an example of how this works. Imagine you have an enormous fish tank with a gigantic fish that is killing all the others. What can you do? You could destroy it by analyzing its speed, size, and habits so that you could calculate the ideal moment to spear it. TCM takes a different approach. Rather than eliminating the enemy, it would add something to the fish's water that would gradually change the entire environment for this particular fish, which, in turn, would control the fish, cause it to perform differently, or make it die.

To illustrate this very important TCM concept of living "with" a particular condition or situation, let's look at two other examples. There is one famous classical herbal formulation for parasites that is many centuries old. This formulation controls the parasite by putting it to sleep rather than killing it. While the parasite still exists within the body, it has been rendered harmless. TCM understands that you can live with a wide variety of conditions as long as they don't bother you. Gallstones are another example. Ancient herbal formulations have been used, again for many centuries, to alter the body's internal Qi and environment so that the gallstone symptoms can be eliminated (not suppressed). Although the patient might experience some occasional mild pain, he or she would benefit tremendously from saving the organ itself. TCM still treats gallstones this way today. Why is the gallbladder so significant? The *Nei Jing* considers it an indispensable organ because its job is to manage or control the function of all eleven other organs. Its meridian is the only one that has an energy connection with the other eleven as well. TCM considers this organ to be the seat of decision making. Because of the nature of the gallbladder's function, a missing one may eventually lead to Alzheimer's disease.

A knowledgeable, classically trained TCM doctor will formulate herbal remedies to accomplish at least three things: help relieve or control the condition's symptoms, address the root cause of the condition as diagnosed, and deliver the right combination of herbs to protect and strengthen the organ(s) that the condition may affect next. A good TCM doctor will never use herbs to cover up or suppress symptoms.

Combining TCM herbs is an art form that cannot be learned from a medical textbook. It is important to understand that combining many herbs in one formula (such as ginseng, *Gingko biloba,* black cohosh) may only give you the benefits of each individual herb. The effect is not always additive. In fact, these modern "miracle combinations," because they are not based on comprehensive herbal theory, have the potential to cause a number of problems. My patients usually enjoy this analogy. I tell them, "Consider how many times Hollywood combines a famous director and a beautiful movie star; just putting them together is no guarantee of a box office hit!" Or, "Look at the world of computers. It would be nice if a PC worked with a MAC, but even if they're made compatible, you can still experience problems." Much of the inspired knowledge about TCM herbal formulations has been passed from master to student over many generations. During my lifetime, I have been privileged to receive this kind of knowledge from several extraordinary masters. Remember too, that herbal treatments are also Qi treatments. It is the essence or Qi, not the scientific properties, that heal.

TCM treatments are not "quick fixes." Jolting the body into good health is, of course, not the way it works. Any TCM treatment takes a little time to have its full effect, because you are trying to correct the root cause. But you should begin to experience some benefit from herbs within a month of treatment. If you don't, something isn't right. Your body is not receptive to the Qi of the herbs, and you need to talk with your herbalist or TCM practitioner, or perhaps find another.

There are a number of herbs being marketed now for menopausal symptoms. Many of them, however, relieve (or simply cover up) symptoms without dealing with their root cause. The principle behind the use of Chinese herbs for menopausal symptoms is to treat their source—the purpose is different. So be careful about the claims made for herbs. Even if your symptoms go away, it doesn't mean you've fixed the root cause or that you've been cured.

There are several Chinese herbs available in capsule form that are particularly good for menopausal women; they are safe to take, and don't require a prescription. One is *dong quai*. (Many Western women going through menopause take this herb, but often don't see enough benefit. I usually recommend that my own patients slowly double the recommended dose on the label for a better result.) Used along with ginseng, it is very helpful in relieving hot flashes. *Dong quai* is good for the blood, and ginseng is good for Qi. Because Qi and blood are an inseparable pair and depend on each other's support, combining these two herbs will give you more benefit than using them alone. Another good herb for menopausal women is *Gingko biloba*, although you must be careful to purchase a quality product.

As I said at the beginning of the chapter, the best treatment is individualized treatment. But this book is about self-healing, and generally speaking there are effective ways to address the common problems experienced by many women. So as I've mentioned earlier, I've adapted several herbal formulas for Western menopause symptoms that address their root cause. They are designed to do two things: boost kidney Qi and strengthen liver function. *Imperial Qi* helps strengthen kidney function; *Green Dragon* goes directly to the liver to help make it function better. These herbal formulas are intended to reinforce organ function so that your own healing ability can take over the job of alleviating your symptoms. Both are based on ancient formulas for Menstrual Cycle Ending Symptoms in use for centuries that I've adapted to address our stressful Western lifestyles. These classical Chinese herbal formulas for menopause can be ordered by contacting our Foundation through the information found at the back of the book.

As my patient, I would, of course, deal with your problem in an individualized way. Depending on your condition, I might tell you that it needed a special herbal formula that I would create from the many drawers and jars of dried herbs in my office. These herbs you would take home and cook into a tea or broth. After analyzing your symptoms, your TCM herbal formula might break down like this:

-50 percent for the liver
-10 percent for symptom prevention
-10 percent for the specific menopausal symptom(s)
-10 percent for the kidney
-5 percent to guide the herbs to their proper organs
-5 percent to test whether the formula is working correctly

Acupuncture

Acupuncture is based on Meridian Theory. It works from the outside, stimulating the meridians or energy pathways in the body. It goes directly to function problems, and helps tune up the body's whole energy system, relieving blockages of Qi, and improving its flow. Acupuncture is helpful in relieving symptoms, but is not powerful enough on its own to get to the root of a problem. Herbs are often used along with acupuncture, for a faster and more complete cure.

There are more than 360 acupuncture points in the body. Out of these, there are roughly sixty main points in the extremities, which can be narrowed down further to a total of eight primary points in the hands and feet. Your acupuncturist must know which points to use, and must be able to hit these points exactly. The best practitioner will use the fewest needles. If a problem can be fixed with two needles, why use ten?

More important than the number of needles is their placement. From my training with many Qigong masters, I believe that needles should never be placed in the following points: *Mingmen* (in the small of the back), *Guanyuan* (a few inches below the navel), *Dazhui* (on the seventh cervical vertebra), *Tanzhong* (in the sternum between the two nipples) and *Baihui* (on the top of the head). These are powerful points for increasing Qi. With most acupuncture points, if the acupuncturist does something wrong, he or she can't do too much harm. That is not the case with these points. If a practitioner has not been properly trained, he or she might actually decrease your Qi by putting a needle in them—or worse, destroy your energy function altogether. Heating these points is a safe way to stimulate them, for instance, by means of a moxibustion stick (a cylinder made from special herbs, lit at one end, with its heat applied to the acupoint). To stimulate *Guanyuan* and *Mingmen,* you can also use an herbal heating pad. (You can find directions for preparing this kind of pad in Recipes for Healing.)

While the placement of needles is more important than how many are used, more important still is the quality of the practitioner's Qi—who is putting the needles in your body. The Qi exchange between doctor and patient is more direct with acupuncture than with herbs; the acupuncturist has to know how to use his or her needles to harmonize a patient's Qi. Acupuncture needles open the body's energy gates to Universal energy. A practitioner not only has to know when, where, and how to use needles, but has to have a feeling for and skill with Qi that goes beyond book knowledge. If your practitioner is just following a recipe—using a book to tell him or her what point to use for what condition—you may not get the most benefit from your acupuncture treatment.

The meridians, as we have seen, play a key role in moving Qi through the body. These pathways form the energy network that connects all internal and external structures. When I explain the concept of meridians, I compare them with the meridians that we see on globes of the earth. Everyone knows that these are not visible lines that you can actually see from the ocean or from the air. Yet, they are critical pathways that allow for ships and airplanes and other navigation-dependent vehicles to pinpoint locations with accuracy. The meridians in your body work in much the same way.

Needles or heat (in the case of moxibustion) are used to relieve a Qi blockage at certain key acupoints to help the body's Qi flow smoothly. They also can be used to readjust an organ's function to achieve harmony inside the body. Some health conditions respond very well to acupuncture; some respond to moxibustion. Some conditions do not respond to either or even both. Again, the well-trained TCM doctor will know when and how to apply each of these specific treatments.

Sometimes, patients say that acupuncture has not helped them. This doesn't mean that acupuncture doesn't work. Acupuncture might not be appropriate for their condition. Their acupuncturist may not be skillful enough to treat their problem, or the acupuncturist's Qi cannot match with their own Qi. For example, pain can come from two causes: external forces like a sports injury or car accidents, among other things, or, pain can come from an internal Qi deficiency or Qi stagnation, such as migraine or allergy headaches, menstrual cramps, arthritis, or chronic lower back or neck pain. Because the cause is different, the treatment should be different as well.

External pain conditions are fairly easy to treat and usually produce benefits quickly. Internal conditions of pain are actually quite complicated and require more knowledge to treat. This is because, unless the root cause is identified, the practitioner may only succeed in relieving symptoms and the risk of the pain recurring remains.

As an example, I have a patient, Sarah, who has had lower back pain for years. When we first met she told me that she had been to many acupuncturists. A friend of hers referred her to me because of our successful relationship in treating her lower back pain in a very short time. Sarah told me that in the past the first few treatments usually relieved her pain, but then it would return. When I asked her how these acupuncturists had diagnosed her, she said that no one had done a four-part diagnosis. No one had asked her about herself and her emotions and her lifestyle habits. Nor did these practitioners spend very much time with her. They put her in a room for thirty minutes with acupuncture needles in the areas where she indicated she had pain, then sent her on her way. She would feel some relief after these treatments, which gave her hope that acupuncture could eventually cure this problem. But always the pain returned within one or two days, sometimes even the same day.

During our first appointment, I told her that I would do my best to help her, but that she needed to realize that because I was able to help her friend's lower back pain, did not necessarily mean that I could help hers. Her friend's lower back pain was caused by a car accident. Because she had no external injury, I told her I believed her chronic back pain pointed to an internal cause.

During my diagnosis, I found that Sarah's pain was related to a kidney Qi deficiency. I could also tell that she had liver Qi stagnation. Her whole body always felt cold, and she suffered from urinary frequency. Her lower back pain was particularly acute during her menstrual cycle, when Sarah also suffered from severe cramps. All these symptoms helped me recognize the source of her problem. Within four treatments, she told me she had about 80 percent ongoing relief from pain. I advised her that complete healing would come from strengthening her kidney Qi and that she needed to conserve her energy for healing by eating foods to boost her kidney Qi (walnuts, scallions, and others listed in Chapter 15) and resting.

Highly trained TCM doctors practice energy acupuncture, which, again, is a technique that cannot be learned from medical texts. Energy acupuncture includes deep insight into what has caused the health problem, as well as into what organs and areas are affected. It also involves knowing how to transfer and add healing Qi to the patient's via acupuncture needles. As we've seen with the above story, putting needles where there is pain without proper and deep diagnosis may create some benefits. But, this is not the true, powerful TCM acupuncture of the ancients. Remember that it is the knowledge, skill, and Qi level of the acupuncturist that makes acupuncture work, not just the needles or the acupoints.

Even though acupuncture has been used to treat pain and many other conditions in China for several thousands of years, it became known in the United States in the early 1970s. Today, the FDA estimates that more than $500 million a year is spent on treatments involving acupuncture and that Americans are now making between nine and twelve million visits annually to practitioners. One very positive advance for acupuncture therapy was the acceptance by the NIH in November 1997 as an effective treatment for postoperative dental pain, nausea, and vomiting caused by anesthesia, chemotherapy, or pregnancy. Another was the reclassification of acupuncture needles by the FDA from experimental medical devices to the same regulated category as surgical scalpels and hypodermic syringes.

Moxibustion

As described earlier, moxibustion uses a stick of compressed herbs that is lit and used to apply heat over a specific meridian or to a specific acupoint to relieve a Qi blockage or to generate Qi.

Generally speaking, any kind of symptoms relating to excess cold, like the common cold, or conditions of internal cold like menstrual cramps, or bed wetting can be helped by moxibustion. This kind of treatment is also good for menopausal symptoms like hot flashes, night sweats, urinary frequency, vaginal discharge, among others. Moxibustion is particularly good for breast cancer patients because of its ability to help dispel cancer's cold yin Qi and generate additional Qi. As with acupuncture, moxibustion should be practiced with the same deep understanding.

Acupressure

Classical TCM acupressure is called *Tuina*. It is the use of special hand techniques or tools to stimulate meridians or acupoints. Although the techniques are different, acupressure is as effective as acupuncture. For some conditions, acupressure is more useful and easier on the patient. For example, sports injuries such as tennis elbow or simple sprains respond better to acupressure. Sometimes acupressure and acupuncture together can accelerate healing benefits. *Tuina* requires more physical strength, more study, more training, and more technical skill than acupuncture. In China, in colleges and universities of TCM, there are separate majors—one for acupuncture, one for acupressure. Even in TCM hospitals, a patient will be directed to two separate departments for treatment. Acupressure is a medical treatment and is not the same as body massage. It is an excellent treatment to help women relieve stress and rebalance their Qi.

Qigong

Qigong is the foundation of TCM. TCM's major theories—Five Element, Meridians, and Organs' Function, Qi and Blood, Yin/Yang—are a result of insight discovered during Qigong practice by ancient TCM doctors. This explains why all famous ancient TCM doctors were Qigong masters. Qigong can do what no other medicine can: help your body, mind, and spirit to connect with each other and function in harmony. It has the power to reawaken and strengthen your body's innate healing ability, and lets you reconnect with the healing Qi of the Universe. Qigong is the best medicine; it is also the most difficult and the most dangerous.

Besides TCM, Qigong also is firmly embedded in Chinese culture and is the foundation of all the Chinese arts, including the fine arts and martial arts. There are many Qigong systems, based on a variety of principles, but essentially Qigong is learned in two ways: by form, or by message. In a Qigong system based on forms or techniques, you learn a variety of exercises, and the emphasis is on doing these exercises correctly. If you do them right, you can increase your Qi; if not, you won't get the benefit. In a message system, you may also learn certain forms, but the essence of the practice is the message transferred to you by the master. If you perform the forms poorly, you'll still get the benefit.

Qigong is something that needs to be taken very seriously. It is not merely an exercise like aerobics. It is not like yoga either. Qigong affects the circulation of all the Qi, or life force, in your whole body. Doing Qigong incorrectly can hurt you. And by the time you find out you've been harmed by your practice, it may be too late to do anything about it. Practiced improperly, Qigong can mix up your internal Qi. It can send your Qi the wrong message, and deflect it from its natural course. Once this happens, it is very hard to fix. If you experience uncomfortable side effects from your practice, such as stomachaches, headaches, insomnia, nightmares, or menstrual disorders, you should stop practicing immediately and discuss your experience with your master. Symptoms like these indicate a Qi imbalance, and you may need to adjust your practice or find another system.

The key to any Qigong practice is a good teacher. You need to find an understanding teacher; this is much more important than a famous teacher. You want someone who will care about you, and who can really help you heal yourself. Qigong has to do with invisible things, not with forms that you can see. In choosing a teacher, you have to use your intuition. If you don't have access to a Qigong school, there are many self-teaching Qigong books and videos available. It's difficult to know which ones are worthwhile.

Some masters can teach by video, some cannot. In order to be able to teach successfully by video, a master has to be able to transmit his or her Qi over a long distance. He or she also has to have some cultural basis in Qigong practice, and a feeling for the dynamics of Qi. Many teachers follow an Eastern practice, but their ideas are still Western. So choose carefully. Put aside all that you may know about Qigong, or the reputation of a particular teacher, and go by your heart.

It is difficult to say how old the practice of Qigong is. Some believe it goes back much further than five thousand years. The word Qigong literally means "energy work," but the actual practice is far deeper than its description. It is a powerful self-healing discipline that is particularly effective for women who want to prevent or alleviate menopausal symptoms. As we've said, Qigong can help you connect your body, mind, and spirit by allowing you to gain control of and direct your own Qi. Its biggest benefit is that it can develop your intuition and let you understand the world in a different way. This view is one that can take you beyond your five senses.

There are several distinct Qigong traditions: Taoist, Confucian, Buddhist, martial arts, and medical. It is this last form of Qigong that is beginning to attract a great deal of attention from Western audiences. I say "beginning" because Qigong was suppressed during the Chinese Cultural Revolution, which lasted from about 1965 to 1976. Qigong, however, never died out in practice; around 1978, it began its rise in popularity again in China. Today, it is estimated that more than 70 million Chinese practice some form of Qigong daily. More and more people around the world are becoming interested in this ancient energy practice. In 1988, the Chinese held the first world conference for showcasing Qigong medical research. Over the past decade, these conferences have grown more popular and are now held every few years.

Qigong is one of the most powerful prescriptions a TCM doctor can use because it works directly on the body's energy system. It is not uncommon in China for women to recover from breast or other kinds of cancer by practicing Qigong, which, is routinely

TRADITIONAL CHINESE MEDICINE

prescribed in TCM hospitals and medical centers. I have worked with my own master on clinical workshops for women with breast masses or tumors at hospitals in China. During these events, we saw immediately that some women were able to reduce or eliminate their masses after just one practice session of *Wu Ming* Meridian Therapy Qigong.

Qigong is an ideal prescription for some of my patients and their particular problems. I often teach my patients one or two simple Qigong movements to help them reawaken their healing ability and to speed up their healing process. This is good for them since the ability to heal themselves is now placed in their hands. They now have something to rely on to heal themselves should the same problem recur. Qigong is particularly good for healing problems that Western medicine cannot identify; frequently these are function disorders that do not show up on scientific tests. This ancient energy practice is particularly effective for healing chronic health conditions as well as specific Qi imbalances and deficiencies like those of menopause. Qigong is also very good for helping correct immune system disorders and chronic conditions of many kinds.

In China, medical practitioners have found that Qigong is effective in treating a wide variety of health conditions, including drug abuse and obesity. In hospitals and clinics across China, Qigong is routinely prescribed to treat arthritis, asthma, bowel problems, diabetes, migraines, hypertension, rheumatism, neuralgia, stress, ulcers, and many others. As we have discussed, Qigong has also been used to successfully treat cancers and reduce or even eliminate debilitating side effects of radiation and chemotherapy. It also can bring special relief to those suffering from chronic pain, and other chronic conditions that affect the digestive, respiratory, nervous, and cardiovascular systems.

Qigong practice has been documented to speed recovery from surgery and sports and other kinds of injuries. I have had great success with prescribing Qigong for a number of patients to help them recover more rapidly from serious injuries, like those of car accidents.

Some of the amazing things that Qigong can do are: strengthen the immune system, lower blood pressure, adjust pulse rates, help alter metabolic rates, adjust oxygen demand, harmonize endocrine system functions, regulate some of the body's basic building blocks, and even slow the process of aging. Above all, the Qigong practitioner learns through her own experience that there is no separation between the body and the mind.

In China, there are thousands of Qigong systems; some are ancient systems passed along for many generations. Some are "instant systems" created by modern masters. Today, very few Qigong systems have been seen or taught in the United States. In my Center in New York, I teach Taoist *Wu Ming* Qigong which traces its lineage back to the ancient masters *Lao Tzu* (6th century B.C.) and *Chuang Tzu* (4th century B.C.). Each Qigong system works differently: some are easy to learn, but deliver few benefits; some are difficult to learn and the benefits are difficult to achieve; some are difficult to learn, but yield great benefits. I believe the best Qigong system should be easy to learn and should allow you to achieve great benefits.

Generally speaking, Qigong systems fall into two categories. Systems in the first category are based on postures and movements that stimulate your internal Qi to help heal yourself. In this case, the practitioner must follow the master's directions precisely to gain any benefits from the system. Results depend on correct posture, how much time you practice, and how well your master can teach. In this system, the connection to posture and getting it correct is more important than the relationship between student and master. With this type of system, the benefits are in proportion to the amount of personal effort you put into the practice.

The second category uses movements and postures, but in a different way. They are used to guide the power of the "energy message" in a particular system from master to student. Doing the forms or postures correctly is not overly important—they are merely "the vehicle," or "transportation," for getting the energy message from master to student. (The concept is similar to using acupuncture needles as a communications vehicle to move Qi from the TCM practitioner to the patient. The success of the treatment depends on who uses the needle.) The student then uses this message to help restore and reenergize the function of his or her internal Qi.

The first type of Qigong is like having your computer professor teach you how to write a program that can help improve your health. Using his instructions, you must write your own program and then use it by yourself in your personal computer. There are no other connections. How well you can apply this program now depends on you and your own intuition. With the second type of Qigong, the professor first reveals to you the principles and theories of the entire health program; he teaches you how to apply this knowledge and how to write your own special program. Then instead of making you do the work of writing the computer program, he surprises you with a gift. He transfers a copy of a first-rate, time-tested program to you, and then allows you to link your own personal computer to the mainframe where all the knowledge of this health program is stored. In this latter system, the energy connection between master and student is more important than postures. Using this kind of program saves enormous energy, which can then be directed toward self-healing.

This type of Qigong is very special because the master can use any object to pass healing energy and messages to his or her patient. For instance, they can give a gift which carries this kind of message. The patient can then wear the gift, like a ring or necklace, and receive additional healing benefits. The master can also use art, like painting, drawing, or calligraphy. In this case, the master will give the patient a special piece of art to take home and use for meditation. Sometimes, a highly skilled master can use music for healing. This music is not like "New Age" meditation music, because when the master creates it, healing energy is basically "channeled" through him or her for a very specific healing purpose, or even for a specific person and condition.

Sadly, it is very difficult to find this kind of Qigong master today. From my experience, it's also difficult to find patients with an open mind who can accept this type of energy treatment. If however, the patient can open her mind, she will encounter the highest level of healing possible. Now, she is being treated directly through healing Qi that reaches deeply into her body and mind. If she's treated with herbs, or acupuncture or acupressure, a transfer vehicle or process is involved. When that happens, just like a battery, there is an automatic step down or reduction in the percentage of the Qi or energy transmitted. Also, this type of treatment requires that the practitioner and patient form a deep energy bond. If you are learning Qigong by message, your heart should become empty to receive the benefit of this practice.

Why are these kinds of Qigong masters hard to find? First these masters must have been taught by a skilled master. Their master must have trained them to discover this special gift. Second, even if they are lucky enough to meet a high-level Qigong master, if they haven't been born to receive this gift, then the gift will never go beyond these masters. This concept becomes more clear when you think about how parents wish their child could inherit their own gift. Most parents would like to pass along their special talents to their children. But, even if a parent is a brilliant musician, they cannot make their child into one. The child has to have both the innate talent and the ability to receive the parent's gift. This gift is beyond technique and beyond words. In its simplest terms, it is an energy transfer.

The *Wu Ming* Meridian Therapy for menopause in this book falls into the second category of Qigong. In Chapter 13, I have selected a set of eight Qigong movements that can help stimulate your Qi to flow freely in the meridians that affect your liver and kidney. They can also help you reawaken your natural healing ability. Remember, the more you practice, the more you will gain.

Chinese Psychology

TCM understands that balanced emotions are essential to well-being. As I explained earlier, specific excessive emotions can cause the function of their corresponding organs to fall out of balance. If an illness is diagnosed as being caused by emotions, TCM believes that the best way to heal its root cause is to counter it with emotions. This seems logical enough, but has almost disappeared in practice.

Here's what we've learned about the organs: The five major organs—liver, heart, spleen, lung, and kidney—are paired with their respective emotions—anger, joy, worry, or overthinking, sadness, or grief, and fear or fright. And, as we've seen, each organ has two different relationships with the other organs: generation and control. In Chinese psychology, the dynamic of control is the useful one. Here's a simple example: the liver controls the spleen. Because the liver's emotion is anger, its emotion naturally has control over the spleen's emotion, which is worry. This dynamic holds true for the other organs and their related emotions. Worry can be used to control fear. Fear can control happiness. Happiness can control sadness. Sadness can control anger. The chart below will give you a better understanding of how TCM relates organs and emotions.

ORGANS	EMOTIONS	CONTROLS	ORGANS	EMOTIONS
Liver	Anger	→	Spleen	Worry
Heart	Joy	→	Lung	Grief
Spleen	Worry	→	Kidney	Fear
Lung	Grief	→	Liver	Anger
Kidney	Fear	→	Heart	Joy

Here are some famous ancient classical examples of psychology treatments I've selected to give you a better idea of how this principle works.

FEAR FIXES EXCESS HAPPINESS

The ancient doctor known as the "King of Psychology" is Dr. Zhang Zi He (A.D. 1156–1228). One day, a patient came to him in desperation because he suffered from a condition of excess happiness. He could not stop smiling; his sleep was now disrupted, and he laughed constantly. He begged the doctor to treat him. Because of Dr. Zhang's reputation, the patient hoped he could be cured. After agreeing to take the case, the doctor checked his patient's pulse and suddenly had a sharp intake of breath. This sharp sound immediately alarmed the patient and made him think that his condition was quite serious. Dr. Zhang then told the patient that he had to leave to search for a very special herb. He left the patient immediately and did not return for several days.

During this time, the patient became increasingly worried. Finally, he became convinced that he was so sick that he was going to die that he started to cry because he thought his condition was hopeless. He told his family that he would not be with them for very long. "My condition cannot be cured. I am certain that I'm going to die," he told them. When the doctor learned that his patient had reached this stage, he returned. He then reassured the patient that his condition was not as serious as he had first thought. He gave him a simple herbal combination and sent him on his way. The problem was cured quickly.

When Dr. Zhang talked with this patient, he understood that the root cause was emotional in nature. He then used the technique of deliberately creating fear to relieve the condition of excess happiness to help the patient recover. In other words, he had used the kidney's emotion to control the excess of the heart's.

HAPPINESS FIXES SADNESS

One lady-in-waiting in the Emperor's court had just heard that her father had been killed by thieves. She became so sad and cried so deeply that no one could console her. After her tears stopped, she began to feel a chest pain. Every day this pain grew worse.

A few months later, it appeared that a small ball or mass had gotten stuck in her chest. Many doctors tried to treat her. No one could relieve her pain. Her family turned to Dr. Zhang and pleaded for his help. He came and immediately started to leap into the air, singing wildly, praying and dancing around like a medicine man. Everyone was startled. This was totally *unexpected and unusual behavior for the famous and dignified doctor.*

Because his movements were so silly and out of place, the lady-in-waiting could not help herself when she saw such crazy things. At first, she started to smile; then, she began to laugh uncontrollably. A few days later, the Qi stagnation that had created the lump, which was really a ball of Qi, under her chest wall was completely relieved. Again understanding the root cause of the physical problem, the doctor was able to use joy to overcome grief.

ANGER RELIEVES ANXIETY OR WORRY

A woman was separated from her merchant husband for several years because he had to travel far away on business. After some time, she began to worry about him constantly. She lost her appetite; she began to stay inside her home and never come out. She lost weight. Her family became very alarmed at her deteriorating condition. They asked many doctors to take her case. Each doctor tried his best to treat her with a wide range of special herbal formulas. None could bring back her appetite and she continued to lose weight until finally she became dangerously ill. One day, Dr. Zhang passed through her town and her family begged him to help. When he found out the original cause of the woman's problem, he suddenly told the woman, "Why are you so upset over this man? I just heard he has found a very rich woman and plans to marry her."

Once the woman heard this, she became so angry that she broke several dishes and stormed out of her house. A few hours later, she returned and still angry shouted: "I'm so stupid. How could I have wasted my love and energy on such a bad man." Then her appetite came back and she started to eat again. She began to recover her health. On his return through her village, Dr. Zhang apologized to her and said: "I'm so sorry. I made such a bad mistake. The man I thought was your husband has the same last name as your husband and even comes from the same region. I hope you will forgive me." Dr. Zhang had used the technique of creating anger to resolve anxiety.

The Right Emotions Can Heal Deep Physical Problems

Here's a contemporary story you might find interesting. One of my patients suffered from chronic fatigue syndrome for ten years along with uterine fibroids. She had dealt with menstrual cycle disorders for many years as well. When she first came to see me, we were both pleased with her healing and saw some excellent results. Everything was coming back into balance and her chronic fatigue was almost gone. This woman ran her own business in the fashion industry. Whenever her busy season arrived, she came under great stress and, unfortunately, her symptoms reappeared.

Because we had built up a good relationship over time and she trusted me, I told her that we had finally reached the deepest part of the problem—her own emotions were dragging her down when her Qi became low, which it did during her most important business cycles. I told her she was holding a lot of sadness and even some anger deep inside. I said, "If you can let this go, you will finally feel much better." I would often joke with her that the answer to her problem would be finding a true love. Many times, I would tell her, "Too bad, I can't create this kind of special medicine just for you!"

Two months later, she returned for her regular tune-up. When I took her pulse, I immediately saw that it had changed significantly. The aura around her face, as well as the energy coming from her face had changed. Even her fibroids had shrunk. She told me that her body was making major changes. I told her, "You must have found the right medicine. You must have fallen in love!" When I asked her what had happened, she said that she met a new lover and that she felt that finally she had found a soul mate. I told her that real love can change everything and that this shift of emotions could truly and deeply heal her health issues for good.

The next section begins with a series of self-healing TCM checklists. They relate to six aspects of your lifestyle: eating, sleeping, work, emotions, pleasure, and frequent discomforts. Be sure and answer the questions. You may be very surprised at the answers.

TO SUMMARIZE:

- For a TCM practitioner, everything about a patient is unique.
- TCM treatment principles are: Treat the root cause; strengthen the body's immune system; harmonize the function of the body's organs; adapt treatment to the specific needs of the individual: "who you are" (body type, genetics), "where you are" (geographical location), "how you are" (physical condition and lifestyle) and "when you are" (age, time of day and season, time of symptom);
- When a new patient comes to see me, I always ask him/her to fill out a TCM Personal Self-Healing Evaluation Form;
- The TCM exam is made up of four diagnostic methods: looking (at the face, eyes, tongue, etc.); smelling and hearing; asking (questions and answers); and touching (including pulse diagnosis);
- Once the TCM practitioner makes a diagnosis, there are several healing tools that can be applied in creative ways: foods, Qigong, herbs, acupuncture and moxibustion, acupressure, and Chinese psychology.

PART THREE

HOW YOU CAN UNLOCK TCM'S ANCIENT SECRETS FOR A NATURAL, HORMONE-FREE MENOPAUSE

CHAPTER 11

GETTING STARTED:
How Healthy Are You?
Test Yourself with These
TCM Checklists

OUR bodies are born with an innate intelligence that governs our ability to self-heal. Our self-healing process is fueled by Qi. If your Qi is strong and balanced, and you take good care of yourself, your own energy system will, by and large, be able to regulate itself. By middle age, however, our bodies are showing the effects of years of stress, possibly unhealthy lifestyle habits, and our Qi has declined and gotten out of balance.

If you are in perimenopause, your body's Qi and the function of your organs are just starting to decline. At this early stage, it may be easy to tune up your system. Acupuncture or herbs, alone or in combination, might well bring quick relief from any symptoms. If they do, be sure not to stop treatment too soon. Even if your symptoms seem to have disappeared, the function of your organs will still need support. It's a good idea to continue treatment for a while so you can be sure you've addressed the source of the problem. If you're taking herbs, for example, keep taking them even if you seem fine. These herbs are designed to help your organs function better so that you can heal yourself. Then you can gradually switch from herbal therapy to self-healing with foods, Qigong, and meditation.

If you're fully into menopause and experiencing its many discomforts, you can now understand where they come from and why. I strongly recommend a healing program that includes both classical Chinese herbs and acupuncture, and some form of energy practice such as yoga, Taiji, or Qigong. This will help unite your body, mind, and spirit. If you're fairly healthy, and the quality of your treatment is good, you should see an immediate improvement in symptoms such as hot flashes, night sweats, and palpitations. If you don't, you should talk to your TCM practitioner to see if your treatment needs to be adjusted. You should discuss whether your symptoms come and go during your treatment, or if they get worse. Even if you do get quick relief from your symptoms, healing their root cause takes longer, at least three to five months. It depends upon your general health, and the skill of your doctor.

If you're not very healthy, your treatment could take up to a year. You must be patient. One thing to remember is that once you've healed the root problem, you will not need herbs or to take acupuncture for the rest of your life. You will have made a successful transition and should be able to make enough estrogen to keep your body healthy for the rest of your life.

As you enter menopause, remember that you now have the last great opportunity to become truly healthy for the rest of your life. I urge you to take responsibility for your own health and healing. It's not up to your doctor to fix you. If menopausal symptoms return, look to your daily lifestyle. Usually this means your everyday habits are still not balanced enough to help you heal yourself thoroughly. Try to find out why your own energy support system is not functioning as it should. You may not be eating well, for example, or you may be working too hard or too many hours. You may not have a peaceful heart. You may also be trying to cope with too much stress. All of these things can consume too much Qi—just at the time when you need to conserve it the most.

If you feel better, you may do what many of my Western patients do. They are so happy to feel well again that they immediately try to go back to their old life, the one they had before their menopausal symptoms slowed them down! Soon, they're spending more Qi than they should. Soon, we're back together again. I say to them, "I don't understand this. Why are you trying to go back to the lifestyle that caused your symptoms in the first place?" Without the resiliency and recuperative powers of a younger body, I tell my patients, "You've got to do things differently now."

So many of my patients say "What should I eat? What should I do to get better? Should I join a gym? Should I start a workout program? How can I get more energy?" I tell them, "I have one secret formula that I've made up for Western women only: do nothing!" They say, "I want to do something." Again I repeat, "Do nothing. That is the best 'something' you can do." My patients laugh and tell me, "You are really something. You have a lot of courage telling Western people that they ought to do nothing, especially in New York City." I will continue to say these things, because they're true. This is the greatest way to heal and live a long healthy life. You are not lazy if you take a rest. You are not lazy if you do nothing. You are being intelligent by conserving your Qi— your body's life force.

SELF-HEALING TCM CHECKLISTS

These checklists are for you. Each one is based on the TCM principles and theories discussed throughout this book. The questions and answers can help you heal yourself and get to a balanced state of health. TCM states that when Qi runs smoothly through the meridians and the organs work in harmony, there is no way for disease or illness to enter your body, not even cancer! Please use these checklists to guide you to new habits and a more healthy lifestyle. If you're in reasonably good health, they can play a major role in helping you reduce or eliminate the discomforts of menopause.

An essential part of a TCM prevention program, these checklists can help alert you to unhealthy lifestyle habits that you should eliminate and minor health problems that you can address to prevent them from becoming catastrophic illnesses, like breast cancer.

Work with these self-healing checklists to create your initial health profile. Copy and fill out the questionnaire in the Appendix. As you perform *Wu Ming* Meridian Therapy, add more healing foods to your diet, and make daily lifestyle changes, you will gradually notice a difference in how well you feel. You will know that this TCM program is having a positive effect. Congratulations! You are beginning to awaken the power to heal yourself!

If you answer yes to more than three of the questions in any one checklist, you should know that your lifestyle can eventually cause you physical problems. These problems will emerge first as a Qi dysfunction. It is critical to understand that if these problems are left uncorrected, they can progress to much deeper physical problems. Don't let this happen to you. Take these signs seriously.

I have set up six separate checklists. Look over the answers and, where possible, try to make the necessary changes they suggest. You can coordinate this knowledge with the *Wu Ming* Meridian Therapy, the energy massage instructions, and the information on healing foods and herbs. With these TCM techniques and tools, you can take control of and responsibility for your healing process.

SELF-HEALING CHECKLIST FOR EATING HABITS: TAKING CARE OF YOUR DIGESTIVE SYSTEM

1. Do you eat barbecued or fried foods often?
2. Do you always drink ice cold drinks or ice water, particularly during your menstrual cycle?
3. Do you eat raw vegetables or eat at salad bars frequently?
4. Do you get a headache after you have a meal?
5. Do you experience stomach distention whenever you eat?
6. Do you have a stomachache after you eat, particularly after eating cold or dairy foods?
7. Do you always burp or pass gas after you eat?
8. Do you always have loose stool after you eat?

9. Do you drink too much alcohol? More than two glasses a day?

10. Do you have food allergies?

Answer Section on Eating Habits

A function disorder of your stomach will cause Qi to stagnate in your stomach meridians. From an energy standpoint, it is essential to keep your stomach functioning well. You should know that 50 percent of breast cancer cases develop in the upper outer quadrant of the left breast, a location TCM understands as being related to the stomach meridian. Therefore, keeping this organ functioning properly is essential to keeping Qi flowing freely in this critical breast area.

1. Barbecued or fried foods can cause a stomach function disorder by creating an excess of heat in this organ. This condition of internal heat can be compared with the kind of heat a compost heap gives off. It is a kind of intense, inner smoldering, which then prevents the stomach from performing its normal job—one aspect of which is to work in harmony with the liver. According to TCM, the stomach and the liver must have a healthy partnership to digest food well. If these two organs cannot work in harmony you will not get enough nutrition or Qi from the foods you eat.

2. The stomach's very nature is warmth-loving. Warmth then is the natural law upon which it operates. Your stomach "loves" to receive warm things like soup, warm drinks like tea, cocoa, etc. If you constantly eat or drink cold foods or beverages, you can unbalance the stomach's natural function and cause it to perform sluggishly. If you frequently eat and drink cold things during your menstrual cycle, your liver and uterus might draw this cold energy to them. This, in turn, can cause cramps, an irregular cycle, or other types of female problems. Try to stick with warm foods and foods with a warm essence.

3. Many people in Western cultures believe that eating raw vegetables provides better nutrition. TCM believes that raw vegetables have a cold essence that can impair the stomach's natural function. Even though you may get a little more nutrition from raw food, you will use up more Qi to digest it. If you cook a vegetable slightly, you may loose a little bit of nutrition, but you will save a lot of Qi that could better be diverted to healing and protecting your stomach function. Because deficient kidney Qi is one of the root causes of menopausal symptoms, it is important to find as many ways as possible to strengthen your Qi. This is something you can do for yourself.

4. Bilateral stomach meridians run up through the forehead area. Generally speaking, headaches in the front of the forehead that occur after a meal indicate a stomach Qi deficiency because the stomach is drawing on too much Qi to digest its food.

5. Stomach distention means that you are suffering from a stomach Qi deficiency. It also indicates that your liver is not working in harmony with your stomach. As we've noted, digesting food well depends on a good partnership between these two organs. Stomach distention means they are not supporting each other's function. Too much stress usually causes this kind of discomfort.

6. As indicated in answer 2, the stomach's nature is warmth-loving. If you get a stomachache after you eat cold foods, your stomach Qi has become unbalanced and is now too cold. This is a signal that you should change your eating habits immediately and switch to giving the stomach warm foods or foods with warm essence (like ginger, cinnamon, scallion, and fennel). Identify the foods and herbs that have a warming essence in Chapter 15. They can help relieve this kind of stomachache.

7. Again, burping or passing gas after you eat indicates that the stomach's Qi is deficient. Your organ does not have enough Qi to manage its assigned task of digestion. If this happens after you eat raw vegetables, cheese or other dairy products, or when you're under stress, it is a sign that your stomach and liver's partnership is shaky. Again, this is a symptom that they cannot function in harmony with each other.

8. Loose stool after eating means that the stomach and spleen both have a Qi deficiency. Your digestive system is weak. Avoid cold foods; substitute warm foods.

9. Excess alcohol will cause the liver's Qi to stagnate. If the liver's Qi stagnates long enough, it will affect the stomach's Qi and cause a disruption in communication between the two organs. Again, here is a lifestyle habit that has the potential to seriously unbalance the harmony between two vital organs. When this happens, your digestive system stops functioning. It then becomes difficult to derive enough Qi and nutrition from any foods you eat to support your body. Most people do not understand that in order for foods, vitamins, nutritional supplements, or even drugs to work in the body, they must be processed by a properly functioning system, which comprises the stomach and the liver. According to TCM, there is virtually no way to extract the proper amount of nutrients you need from whatever you put into your stomach if the processing plant itself is not working.

10. Food allergies are an indication that your stomach Qi is low or deficient. It also means that your stomach cannot work in harmony with the liver, spleen, and gallbladder. Many people, in an attempt to address their allergies, gradually cut out one food after another in their diet in the hope of relief. Sometimes, I see patients who are basically down to eating rice cakes and water because they have become so sensitive. They are so focused on believing that their problem is caused externally by the foods themselves, that they are literally shocked when I tell them it is their stomach that is the problem. Changing your diet alone does not get to the root cause of food allergies. Avoiding cold foods, raw foods, and ice cold liquids can help significantly. Adding warm foods and foods with a warm essence like ginger and cinnamon can also help. Start changing your diet today using the information in this book. If you suffer from food allergies, this step can make a big difference in the state of your health. Practicing *Wu Ming* Meridian Therapy can help by increasing Qi and relieving Qi stagnation.

SELF-HEALING CHECKLIST ON SLEEP HABITS

1. Do you have difficulty going to sleep each night?
2. Do you wake up at the same time each night? What time?
3. Do the same dreams recur frequently?
4. Do you have nightmares?
5. Do you experience night sweats?
6. Do you go to bed after midnight?
7. Do you eat a big meal and then go to sleep?
8. Do you have to take a sleeping pill or other drug to sleep soundly?
9. Do you get up to urinate frequently during the night?

Answer Section on Sleep Habits

Sleep is the natural state in which both your physical body and its energy system take a rest and regenerate themselves. During this time, your body's Qi can recharge itself—much like a battery. If you sleep well, your body is ready to go with a new charge. If you sleep poorly and wake often, you have less Qi to get through your day. TCM examines your dreaming to diagnose the quality of your sleep. For example, if your body is in deep harmony, your sleep will be quite deep, and you should not consciously remember your dreams. You still dream, but these dreams are not accessible to your conscious mind. TCM also uses dream interpretation to understand the condition of the Qi of your various organs.

1. If you have difficulty falling asleep continually, generally speaking, your spleen and heart Qi are deficient. This means these two organs are not functioning in harmony. Remember in our discussion of balance and harmony, we said that the state of harmony reflects one dynamic system which has a smooth, automatic, unconscious exchange of energy. In this instance, your spleen and heart are out of sync. Your heart is not peaceful enough to contain your spirit and you cannot calm down long enough to fall asleep. If you toss and turn during sleep, the cause is the same.

2. TCM theory states that Universal Qi changes every two hours. The Qi in your organs also changes every two hours. Like a giant gear, if your Qi cannot match or mesh with Universal Qi changes, then many different kinds of physical discomforts will develop. TCM recognizes these conditions as biorhythm disorders. For example, Qi changes start with the lung, which is "on duty" or in charge of the body, from 3:00 to 5:00 A.M. If your lung's Qi has a problem, then you might find yourself waking up during this two-hour window. Or, you might wake up with a physical problem like a cough during these hours. Here are the other two-hour periods in which each organ's Qi is in charge:

Lung	3:00 A.M.–5:00 A.M.
Large intestine	5:00 A.M.–7:00 A.M.
Spleen	7:00 A.M.–9:00 A.M.
Stomach	9:00 A.M.–11:00 A.M.
Heart	11:00 A.M.–1:00 P.M.
Small intestine	1:00 P.M.–3:00 P.M.
Bladder	3:00 P.M.–5:00 P.M.
Kidney	5:00 P.M.–7:00 P.M.
Pericardium	7:00 P.M.–9:00 P.M.
Triple warmer	9:00 P.M.–11:00 P.M.
Gallbladder	11:00 P.M.–1:00 A.M.
Liver	1:00 A.M.–3:00 A.M.

3. Dream diagnosis or interpretation is one tool TCM uses to understand a patient's physical condition. Problems that are Qi or energy-related in the internal organs show up in different kinds of dreams. For instance, if your heart Qi is deficient, you might feel yourself falling out of the sky, or off a tall building. If you have a kidney Qi deficiency, you might have dreams that are connected to drowning or being under water, or being in a boat that is capsizing. Or, you might find yourself being fearful and hiding from something in your dreams. If you refer to the Five Element The-

ory chart on page 68, you can see where this insight comes from. Water is the element of the kidney and fear is its ruling emotion. You can gain more insight into your dreams by studying the Five Element Chart. If you always see yourself arguing or fighting or things are destroyed in your dreams, then you might have a parasite, or these could be signals that your internal problem might be worsening.

4. Generally speaking, nightmares indicate a liver Qi deficiency—nightmares that contain images of people chasing you, wanting to kill you, or harm you usually indicate a problem with unbalanced liver Qi. If you have these kinds of nightmares, your physical liver organ may be fine, by the way it is functioning is definitely in need of attention. If these dreams occur frequently, your body is sending you stronger signals that the liver needs your help. According to TCM, the liver is the most important organ for women's health. I recommend that you pay serious attention to these kinds of internal warnings. Remember if Qi stagnates in the liver or this organ becomes completely out of balance, you are looking head on at the root cause of breast cancer.

5. Sweating at night indicates that your body's yin Qi is deficient. This means that at nighttime your body's Qi cannot control the normal opening and closing of your skin pores. One of the key principles of TCM is that the body has two types of Qi—yin and yang—that must work in harmony. Daytime Qi is considered yang; nighttime Qi yin. If you have more physical discomfort in the daytime, your body's yang Qi is deficient or is not sufficient enough to handle normal daytime tasks. The reverse is true if your problems occur at night.

6. Also, if you experience night sweats during chemotherapy, radiation, or tamoxifen therapy, this means that these treatments are having a serious effect on your yin Qi. This is a sign that you should add things like clam juice or oyster juice to your diet. Adding ginseng in any form can also help. Special classical Chinese herbal formulas can stop this problem and help strengthen you through these treatments. These combinations are in widespread use today in China in conjunction with Western-type cancer treatments.

It is important to understand this from a Qi perspective. Your body enters its yin Qi phase after midnight—your body's yang Qi makes its way deep into your internal organs with the goal of rejuvenating them. To remain in harmony, your body should follow nature's way. If you stay up past midnight, you are working against nature's cycle. Your body will spend more than twice the amount of Qi for every hour you're awake just to stay awake. To conserve your Qi and prevent disease or illness, it's important to follow nature's cycle. This is an especially key lifestyle habit to change before you reach perimenopause or menopause. For women undergoing cancer treatments, which, of course, already deplete the body of Qi, you can see why you need to get to bed early and get a good night's sleep.

7. Many people in the United States eat a big dinner and then go to sleep. This often causes sleep problems. TCM understands that insomnia is related to different types of stomach Qi dysfunctions. When you eat a big meal, the stomach's Qi will overfunction or work too hard. By overworking, it can fall out of harmony with the liver and heart. (Refer to the Five Element Chart to see the kinds of relationships these organs share.) That's why some people feel heartburn after a big meal; however, the root cause is often a stomach Qi dysfunction. Healthy eating means that you should only eat 70 to 75 percent capacity of your stomach. Eating too much before bedtime can cause your stomach to use extra Qi to function all night long just to digest what you've eaten, when it should be conserving this Qi for self-healing and resting. Here again is another seemingly simple, yet effective, way where you can build up your Qi for healing during menoapuse and not waste it.

8. TCM understands that sleeping well means your body is functioning in harmony. If you frequently or always rely on sleeping pills or drugs, your body cannot function in harmony. Also, these substances might be hiding a deeper internal problem that needs to be fixed. I recommend that my patients try to find other natural ways to help them sleep better. Celery juice can help with insominia.

9. Urinary frequency during the night indicates a kidney Qi deficiency. This means that your kidney cannot send its partner organ, the bladder, the right messages and enough Qi to hold your urine throughout the night. This problem can appear during menopause and cause fatigue. The eighth Qigong movement in the *Wu Ming* Meridian Therapy series can help you strengthen your kidney Qi. If this condition occurs during or after cancer treatments, it means your body's overall Qi has dropped significantly. If so, I recommend frequent practice.

SELF-HEALING CHECKLIST ON WORK HABITS

1. Do you work in or around high power electrical areas, or where there is radiation, such as a microwave?
2. Do you work with chemicals?
3. Do you like your job?
4. Do you work under chronic stress?
5. Do you work straight through your day without taking a lunch break?
6. Do you work and eat at the same time?
7. Do you get along with the people you work with?
8. Is your work area comfortable and healthy?

Answer Section on Work Habits

Your daily lifestyle has a tremendous impact on the state of your health. Understanding how to shape your work experience so that it supports your health is a very important aspect of self-healing. Many women spend more than eight hours a day at their workplace. While you may not be able to change your workplace itself, you can begin to pay attention to any negative effects it has on you and begin to change your responses to it. I find that many of my patients work very hard to reduce or even eliminate their menopausal symptoms and make this hormone-free transition we've talked about; however, if they do not learn how to change their response to stress in the workplace, they find themselves dealing with the same symptoms again and again.

I remind my patients that it is their old lifestyle that has contributed to their current physical problems. I advise them not to be so eager to "get back to their life." Here is where I urge you to change your habits and your emotional responses to the many stresses in your daily life if you truly want to heal and address the root cause of your menopausal symptoms. Most important, if you want to prevent breast cancer or its recurrence, then you need to understand how to change your daily work habits so they do not deplete your Qi or vital energy.

1. Electrical fields can interfere with or change your body's own electrical field. Recent scientific work with bioelectromagnetics at Stanford University in California shows that even very subtle frequencies, far below what was considered safe previously, can create cellular changes. Electrical fields can cause a dysfunction in the flow of Qi through your meridians. They also have the ability to cause a serious Qi deficiency. The stronger the field, the worse the effect. If you work around areas with a lot of radiation, your energy field can also be easily disrupted and unbalanced by this kind of energy force. If you are continually exposed to these kinds of energies, you are at risk for compromising your own self-healing ability.

2. Certain kinds of chemicals can either directly or indirectly cause cancer. Even if you don't touch the chemical itself, simply smelling it can disrupt the smooth and healthy functioning of your lung. How is this possible? Remember that, according to TCM theory, the sense organ associated with the lung is the nose. Additionally, the lung controls the health of the skin. If your lung function is interrupted, then your skin can be affected.

3. Because you spend the largest part of your day at your job, you invest a lot of emotional, physical, mental, and spiritual energy there. If you don't like your job, but you must keep it, then your mind and spirit are in conflict and under constant pressure. This condition can cause internal Qi stagnation in any organ or meridian. This is the earliest state of an imbalance within the body. It is also related to the root cause of breast cancer.

If you always find yourself in this situation, physical problems will eventually show up somewhere in your body. For instance, during the menstrual cycle, you may experience PMS, headaches, sleep problems, breast tenderness, and so on. As you enter perimenopause or go through the menopause years, continually holding these kinds of negative emotions can aggravate menopausal symptoms. You may not relate these symptoms to chronic emotional distress, but according to TCM theories, this is the root cause of the physical discomfort.

4. Stress takes a deadly toll on the liver, which is the most important organ for women's health. If your liver function is out of balance, then you might experience physical discomfort in the form of symptoms such as menstrual disorders, PMS, stomach distention or bloating, nail problems, and itchy and/or red eyes. If the liver continues to be stressed over time, this condition can lead to function disorders of your other major organs, the stomach, kidney, heart, and lung. It is vital to find a healthy way to deal with the stress in your life. It is important not to absorb the negative energy of stress into your own energy system, but find productive ways to let it go. Remember we discussed menopause as a woman's last great healing opportunity and a doorway to a new way of life. If you live with chronic stress, especially in your job, think carefully about how you can change this health-robbing situation, and, if you cannot, whether you are really willing to give away your health and longevity in return for a paycheck.

TCM has a time-honored and very successful way to alleviate anger: smash eggs! In fact, buy a dozen eggs (a pretty inexpensive way to let out stress) and smash them all. Believe it or not, this simple act can help you physically and emotionally relieve a lot of anger and stress. As I mentioned earlier, many of my menopause patients laugh and say to me, "Why didn't you tell me to buy two dozen eggs! I loved smashing these eggs and I really felt a major energy shift within me by doing this. What an amazing experience." No eggs? Try smashing raw potatoes with your feet (shoes on!). Or, in a safe place, break glass bottles. Releasing negative energy can definitely help you heal the root cause of a number of problems; the results are remarkable.

Acupuncture, Taiji, Yoga, and meditation, as well as certain Chinese formulas can help relieve stress. Our *Wu Ming* Meridian Therapy movements are especially effective at helping you reduce chronic stress in your life. Beyond this, they can also help you deepen your spiritual connection with the Universe and its vibration of unconditional love.

5. Because of the multiple lives women lead, they often work long, stress-filled hours, sometimes forgetting to stop for lunch. This causes the body to burn up extra Qi for daily activity. When this happens, your body is forced to draw on its irreplaceable kidney Qi to keep going. This is not a good situation because we've seen how it should be running instead on the Qi of your rechargeable stomach energy to get through the day. Try to change this habit immediately. Tell yourself that you are entitled to live a healthy life. Find at least fifteen or twenty minutes every day to eat lunch properly.

Not eating healthy foods at regular intervals will cause a stomach function disorder that could eventually lead to digestive system problems later like food allergies, bloating after eating, and weight gain. Again, continuing this unhealthy habit can lead to more serious digestive problems when the stomach becomes unable to extract nutrition from the things you eat. Function problems of the stomach itself or problems of Qi stagnation in the stomach's meridian could disrupt the healthy flow of Qi through the stomach meridians, which run through the breasts. A Qi blockage in this area can lead to the development of a mass or worse.

6. Working and eating at the same time is not a healthy habit. If you make a regular practice of doing this, then your digestive system will not get sufficient Qi to do its job. You may not be able to gain maximum nutrition from the food you're eating while you're working. If you continually work and eat at the same time, you may not know it, but you can literally upset or unbalance the normal healthy functioning of your stomach. Then, one of the problems you may eventually experience is stomachaches after eating. Many women begin to develop digestive problems when they reach menopause. Here is one daily activity that you can change for the better to help yourself heal. Even if it's only twenty minutes, take some time for yourself and eat your meal in peace and quiet. Do not answer the phone, or hold a meeting, or try to balance your checkbook at this time. Just take the time to eat slowly and thoughtfully. Since 50 percent of breast cancers appear in the area through which the stomach meridians run, it is critical to do everything you can to keep this organ and its meridians functioning well. This is true prevention.

7. While you don't have to love the people you work with, it's very important to have a harmonious work experience. Otherwise, your body will spend extra Qi to deal with emotional issues on a daily basis. This emotional discomfort can cause a function disorder of one or more of your five major organs. Go back to the Five Element Theory chart and review which emotions can affect which organs. According to TCM theories, holding unbalanced and/or negative emotions in the body for a long time, can lead to Qi stagnation and cause serious damage.

I want to emphasize that it is not experiencing an emotion that is damaging (unless, of course, it is sudden and severe). We're all human and we experience a range of emotions each and every day. It is chronically holding negative emotions that cause health problems. To remain well, it is important to find productive ways to release excess emotions from your body and become good at "letting things go." Try to follow nature's lead, especially as you enter menopause, and "go with the flow."

8. Again, because you spend so many of your waking hours in the workplace, it is very important to create harmony in your environment to the best of your ability. This way your body does not have to divert extra Qi just to maintain its normal functions. Even a few small changes can help you conserve your Qi. When a plant flowers, it is at the peak of its own Qi. Try to bring a fresh flower into your workspace often to experience this special energy. This kind of "live" message can help your body recall its own healing ability. Place a healthy green plant near your computer. When your eyes become tired, change your field of vision to the plant, and rest it there for a few minutes. This can help you relieve eyestrain and help keep your vision healthy.

Everyone can take a few short breaks throughout the workday. When you do, close your eyes and breathe slowly and deeply. Let everything go; do not focus on any problems or physical sensations or emotions. I tell my patients that even a few minutes done occasionally throughout the day can really help them recharge their energy base. From my experience, many short meditations can produce the same effect as twenty minutes of continuous meditation. Getting into this habit can change your life and help you accumulate tremendous health benefits. Since one of the two major causes of menopausal conditions is declining kidney Qi, imagine how much you can help yourself by taking these moments to strengthen your own Qi.

SELF-HEALING CHECKLIST ON EMOTIONAL STABILITY

1. Do you have depression? Do you take medication for depression?
2. Do you suffer from anger continually?
3. Do you cry easily and often?
4. Do you suffer from anxiety or panic attacks?
5. Is it hard for you to make decisions?

6. Do you worry all the time?
7. Are you under a lot of stress for continued periods of time?
8. Do you suffer from frequent mood swings?
9. Do negative events from the past continue to bother you today?

Answer Section on Emotional Stability

TCM does not believe emotions are an experience that occurs only in your mind or in your thoughts. It identifies five specific emotions that, if experienced excessively, have the ability to destroy the healthy functioning of an organ. As we've seen in the Five Element Theory, TCM believes the liver is related to the emotion of anger—too much anger held for a long period of time can unbalance healthy liver function. Overthinking or constant worry will cause stomach and spleen function problems, sometimes manifesting as a loss of appetite or excess water retention, respectively. Healthy lung function can be destroyed by chronic sadness or grief. A continual state of fear will compromise the kidney's regular function. And too much joy or too much happiness will ultimately cause a heart function problem. If you want to remain healthy as you go through menopause, you must keep your emotions in a state of balance. As you grow older, and the risk of breast cancer rises, it is particularly critical to watch your emotional state. For more than five hundred years, TCM has understood that emotional imbalances are directly related to the root cause of breast cancer.

 1. TCM understands depression as a disharmony between liver and spleen Qi. If you use drugs to help alleviate depression, you may have a temporary lifting of the condition but the underlying root cause is still there. Like pushing a ball under water, sooner or later the problem will pop up again unless this root cause is fixed. TCM understands that treatment of this problem means addressing both the internal Qi imbalances and the emotional reactions to external factors that cause this illness. It is important to identify why and how this problem has come about. Although drugs for depression have helped many people through many difficult times, it is important to recognize that they can eventually cause liver and stomach function problems. They also cannot heal the root cause of depression.

2. Anger will cause a liver function disorder. TCM understands that the liver is the most important organ for women's health. Because the liver is responsible for the smooth flow of Qi and blood throughout the body, a liver function disorder can also cause other organs to become out of balance. If this happens, you might experience menstrual problems such as nausea, cramps, headaches, and breast tenderness during the menstrual cycle. I see a lot of patients who believe they are not angry people and have let their anger over certain situations go. If you ask them if they are angry, they will tell you no. However, when they begin to talk about something that bothers them, they exhibit all the signs of anger, even though in some cases, the event was long ago.

Most women who suffer from menopausal discomforts, have experienced problems with their menstrual cycles for years. If you are a younger woman, you can see how important it is to fix the root cause of your menstrual problems. If anger, or stress, becomes chronic, then the liver's function will deteriorate and Qi can stagnate in the meridian. These are the root causes of breast masses or uterine tumors.

3. Crying is related to the lung function and sometimes the stomach and spleen functions. Crying all the time can weaken the Qi of all three organs. They will then not be strong enough to keep their ruling emotions stable (be sure and identify these emotions from the Five Element Chart), nor will they be able to help keep your overall emotional Qi stable.

4. Anxiety and panic attacks are related to deficient kidney Qi. These conditions can also mean that your kidney and heart are not functioning in harmony. Because the kidney is the Qi

foundation for the entire body, the best way to address these conditions is to treat the root cause by strengthening kidney Qi with classical Chinese herbs.

5. TCM understands that the gallbladder rules the body's decision-making capability. If your gallbladder Qi is deficient, or the gallbladder itself has a function disorder, you might have a hard time making decisions. If your gallbladder has been removed, you might also find—especially as you get older—that making decisions becomes difficult. Even though your physical gallbladder may be removed, remember that its meridian still runs in your body. I remind my patients who have had any organ or organs removed, that they are different now. They must take very good care of themselves to remain healthy. I urge you to do the same.

Sometimes, gallbladder problems are also related to a liver function problem. Remember that these two organs share an energy relationship, that is, they are partners connected via Qi. If you're always under a lot of stress, or if your liver does not function smoothly with this companion organ, or with the other organs, then gallbladder function will be impaired. Also, if you have digestive problems, such as difficulty eating protein or dairy products, the root problem can lie with an unbalanced relationship between the gallbladder and the liver.

6. Constant worry can cause spleen and stomach function disorders. If that happens, your digestive system will be affected. Your body will not be able to extract enough nutrition from what you eat, you might experience lack of appetite, you might retain water, and your sleep may become disturbed. Conversely, if your spleen Qi becomes weak or deficient, you may begin to worry constantly.

7. Stress is the number one external emotional cause of liver function disorder; anger is the number one internal emotional cause. Unfortunately, many women today are affected by both of these conditions. This is especially true of women who reach the age of menopause. They are often in the middle of many "life

events"—from divorce, to children leaving home, to changes in work responsibilities, to the care of an aging or infirm parent, or the death of a parent. If a liver function disorder develops, then you're very likely to have a digestive problem. The consequence of this is an internal Qi crisis. When this crisis occurs, your whole body's energy system can become deficient or weak. The body lacks enough power to support everyday life. It starts "running on empty." This, in turn, causes more stress as you become increasingly unable to manage basic daily activities.

Chronic stress can actually be deadly. It can cause serious Qi stagnation in the meridians and causes most of the health problems many women experience. TCM believes that, for women in transition, as long as kidney Qi can be kept strong and liver function can be kept smooth, then menopausal symptoms can be avoided. Achieving this state can also help address the root causes of breast cancer. That is why I warn my patients that they must examine their lives seriously and try to eliminate stress and anger wherever possible. This is real prevention.

8. If you suffer from frequent mood swings, particularly before your period, or at menopause, or after cancer treatments, two key organs are affected. Your liver Qi is stagnating (the concept of stagnation is like that of a compost heap, which generates a kind of smoldering, internal heat that blocks the free flow of Qi) and your kidney Qi is weak or deficient. Acupuncture and Chinese herbs are very successful treatments for these kinds of problems. Taiji, yoga, meditation, and gaining support from and relating to nature's own Qi by walking slowly and peacefully outdoors can help you regain your emotional balance.

9. As a method of treatment, TCM tries to relieve or unblock Qi stagnation. If you always mull over the past, replay distressful scenes, reflect on past negative events and feelings, hold grudges, or never forgive, sooner or later this stuck Qi, or Qi stagnation, can turn into a physical blockage, like a tumor or cancer. If you want to heal yourself, completely letting things go is the only way to change your body's energy pattern—no matter what problem, the technique is the same. Since liver Qi stagnation is one of the two root causes of menopausal symptoms for Western women, it is important to recognize the health benefits of "letting go."

"Letting go" is one of the most important philosophies of TCM, which uses many different techniques to push disease and illness out of the body. These include treating a cough to expel it from the body instead of suppressing it, or using herbs to put a parasite to sleep instead of trying to eject it with harsh chemicals. And, when it comes to cancer, one of the major TCM treatments involves strengthening the immune system so that it creates an energy field stronger than the cancer itself and within which it can be contained. TCM prefers not to use up the body's finite reserves of Qi to fight head on with the cancer, but rather to focus on helping the patient live a long life—in many cases alongside of the cancer itself. This approach is used successfully in China today to treat cancer patients.

SELF-HEALING CHECKLIST ON PLEASURE HABITS

1. Do you have to be in constant motion?
2. Do you overeat?
3. Do you smoke?
4. Do you drink too much alcohol? More than two glasses per day?
5. Do you have frequent sex or frequently change sex partners?
6. Do you perform high-impact exercises more than three times a week?
7. Do you take drugs, either prescription or recreational drugs?
8. Do you take birth control pills?

Answer Section on Pleasure Habits

1. If you're always in constant motion, you are using up a lot of excess Qi to support your physical and emotional needs. The body is much like a car. It needs a rest; at regular intervals it needs its engine turned off and it needs to cool down. Also like a car battery, the body needs to recharge itself. According to TCM theory, everyone is born with a finite amount of Qi. If you constantly use up large quantities of Qi, it hastens the time when this finite amount is completely depleted; in other words, it's time to die. It may appear that you're accomplishing a lot of things when you're in constant motion, but in reality, you may not be doing the best job, or even the highest quality work. You may be in motion without reason.

If you're one of those people who must be in constant motion, you may also tend to become frustrated more easily. This can unbalance your liver function, which, in turn, can set off a negative cycle that can lead to more serious health problems. When your energy level falls too low or weakens, you are also more vulnerable to getting sick. You do not have an adequate reserve of Qi to heal yourself. Learn to say "enough" and give yourself permission to slow down and make intelligent choices about how to use your time and your Qi. I realize this is particularly hard for women to do because of the many demands placed on them. I have found that many of my patients approaching menopause or going through menopause are reluctant to slow down. They believe that somehow they're lazy or unproductive. Deep down some of them think they will not seem as youthful if they try to make their lives easier. I like to remind them, as I am happy to remind you, that making healthy choices is the most important thing they can do for themselves and their loved ones.

2. If you continually overeat, you can cause a serious stomach function disorder. Your stomach will become distended; you might experience heartburn. Overeating will also cause your body to spend much more of its Qi to digest what you've eaten. According to TCM, a stomach dysfunction can also cause insomnia. Often, sleep problems are caused by eating a big meal too late at night. If you have this kind of problem, don't take sleeping pills. Shift your eating habits and avoid eating or drinking too much before bedtime. Healthy eating means eating enough not to feel hungry later. This requires tuning into your body's signals so that you can recognize what a satisfied feeling means for your body. I recommend my patients eat to about 70 percent of the capacity of their stomach. Not eating too much can also improve your mental function by helping you think more clearly and eliminate a sluggish feeling.

3. Everyone knows that smoking is harmful to your health. Cigarette smoke can not only cause lung cancer by affecting this organ and its meridian, but it will also affect the organs and meridians with which the lung shares an energetic relationship— your large intestine and kidney. Although you may not realize it, smoking can cause large intestine and kidney function disorders. If these two organs are out of balance, you will gain weight after you've quit smoking because both of these organs, which have the job of ridding the body of excess water, have also been thrown out of balance. Remember that the tissue of the lung is the skin. Smoking will also compromise your skin quality.

4. Excessive drinking can cause liver problems. However, according to TCM, the liver has additional and very different functions than it does in Western medicine. For women, if the liver is out of balance, it will affect the stomach's function and cause menstrual cycle disorders and emotional problems. If liver problems continue, you might eventually experience Qi stagnation in the liver meridian, which has a major influence on breast health. Other symptoms of liver Qi disorders include breast tenderness before your periods, headaches on the sides of your head during your menstrual cycle, continual stomach bloating, bad breath, and a red nose (which is due to excess internal heat in the stomach). Drinking a glass of wine occasionally may not harm you, but if

you want to protect your liver and healthy liver function, avoid drinking any alcoholic beverage to excess.

5. In TCM's view, too much sex will cause liver and kidney Qi deficiencies. You might experience a lot of vaginal discharge. If the discharge worsens and becomes yellow or burns and itches as well as takes on a bad odor, you might then experience ringing in the ears, hair loss, and lower back pain. If you really overdo sex, you can even experience eye problems. If you are suffering from menopausal symptoms, you should have sex in moderation until these symptoms are under control. Sex consumes a lot of Qi. Here is another area where you can save your Qi for self-healing. If you are undergoing chemotherapy or radiation, you definitely need to have sex in moderation—for instance, about once or twice a month. Changing sex partners frequently uses up too much liver and kidney Qi and can cause additional female problems. You also might contract a sexually transmitted disease if you do not protect yourself. Naturally, if you have other health problems, this can compromise any effort to self-heal, especially during menopause.

6. Many women have been told that they are doing the right thing by exercising vigorously. They've been told that high-impact exercise will help protect their cardiovascular health. TCM regards exercise differently. First of all, the body is approximately 70 percent water. A water type of body needs water-type exercises to match its energy frequency. Also, TCM theory states that the tendon is the "tissue" of the liver and is governed by this organ. Tendons are like any other structures in the body, they have their limits in terms of function. In this case, a tendon is like a rubber band, you can only stretch it so far and so many times before it loses its elasticity or ability to perform.

High-impact exercises often cause tendon problems that, in turn, can affect the liver and create a liver function disorder. That's why some women who overexercise do not menstruate, or have trouble with their periods. They have developed a liver function disorder that now impedes the free flow of Qi and blood in their body. I see a lot of chronic fatigue syndrome patients—almost all of them have a history of overexercising, especially with high-impact aerobics. I recommend soft exercises like dancing, Yoga, Taiji, and, of course, noncompetitive and gentle swimming, which matches well with our "watery" bodies. One of the best exercises of all is slow, gentle walking in nature, where you can tune up your body, mind, emotions, and spirit with nature's healing Qi. I recommend being fully present in nature—don't wear earphones, don't carry weights, don't speed walk. If you want to test your cardiovascular condition and go beyond the physical level, pay particular attention to the last movement in *Wu Ming* Meridian Therapy. I've challenged a lot of people to stand in this position for more than five minutes. Even if they can run for forty minutes, or stay on a treadmill for an hour, almost no one without practice or training can perform this Qigong movement for more than five minutes. I also challenge you. The longer you hold this posture, the more benefit you will gain, not only for your physical heart and lung, but also for your spirit.

7. If you're a frequent drug user—whether nonprescription or prescription—it's likely that your symptoms are being addressed instead of their root cause. Most drugs are constructed in such a way as to suppress a problem instead of healing its root cause. All drugs are toxic to some degree; they must all eventually be processed through your kidney and liver. For your own health, you need to identify the root cause of your problem instead of continually addressing its symptoms. Because you are a holistic system, sooner or later, the health problem you believe you're treating can emerge in another part of your body. If you're under drug treatment, you can also look for complementary treatments that can help strengthen your Qi, so you might eventually be able to reduce your drug dosage. This way, your immune system can become stronger and can allow your own natural healing ability to take over. Work with your doctor to see what is possible. I've

noticed that many of my menopause patients have doctors that are open to approaching treatment with this in mind.

8. Birth control pills affect the liver, which, as we've stated many times throughout this book, is the most important organ for women's health. TCM believes that unless the liver functions in harmony with your other organs, you cannot get pregnant. To help women who have difficulty getting pregnant, TCM treats the liver and coaxes it back into balance so that it functions smoothly with all the other organs. Because birth control pills suppress your ability to become pregnant, they also suppress your liver function.

Women who have been taking birth control pills for many years often experience difficulty getting pregnant because their liver function has become impaired. Remember here we are not referring to the physical liver. I have helped quite a few women who were infertile become pregnant. When they come to see me, they tell me that they have done all the tests possible and that their liver "is in good condition." I help them understand that while the scientific tests show their organ is all right, my TCM diagnosis shows that the function of their liver is definitely out of balance. When the whole body isn't working in harmony a lot of things can go wrong.

SELF-HEALING CHECKLIST FOR FREQUENT DISCOMFORTS

1. Do you suffer from PMS?
2. Do you suffer from hayfever?
3. Do you suffer physical symptoms when the weather or the seasons changes?
4. Do you frequently have bad breath?
5. Do your ears ring?
6. Are your nails brittle or cracked?
7. Is your nose area red all the time?

8. Do your eyes tear frequently?
9. Do you have frequent headaches?
10. Do you suffer from adult acne?

Answer Section on Frequent Discomforts

1. There is some controversy in the West as to whether or not PMS really exists. TCM has a long history of successful treatment of the complex of PMS symptoms, which it relates to a liver function disorder. PMS has a wide range of associated problems, such as many different types of headaches including migraines, nausea, constipation, loose stool, anger, depression, mood swings, among others. The root cause of all of these seemingly unrelated conditions is the same—liver Qi stagnation. As long as the liver function disorder remains untreated, these problems will remain. I often see patients who regard PMS as simply something they must put up with every month, uncomfortable or, in some cases, debilitating as it is. I really try to educate these women about this condition and what a serious warning sign it is. I urge them to treat the root cause. If they don't they are in for more health problems ahead. Almost always, women with PMS have a difficult menopause.

2. Hayfever usually occurs in the spring and fall. According to TCM, if an organ's energy function cannot match a season's energy change, then you will become sick. Spring is the season of the liver, and the eye is the "window" of the liver. If you get hayfever in the spring, you might have the most trouble with itchy, watering eyes. Fall is the season of the lung, and the nose is its "window." Accordingly, if you get hayfever in the fall, you might experience the most trouble with a runny nose. No matter what season, if your organs are out of balance with Universal energy changes, you will most likely experience some kind of health problem. Fixing the organ's function is the way to permanently address this problem; covering up the symptoms with medications is only a temporary measure.

3. If your body's Qi or energy is not in harmony when weather or seasonal changes occur, your body will produce different kinds of health problems. For example, if your body has too much dampness or maintains a lot of water, then when it's damp or the rainy season comes, you may experience arthritic pain. If you always catch a cold or the flu in the winter, the season that the kidney rules, your condition is related to a kidney Qi deficiency. If you experience headaches at the top of your head or excessive anger or mood swings when winter turns to spring, your liver function is out of balance. If you have heart problems or heart disease, you might experience a lot of discomfort in the summer whose ruling organ is the heart. Women in transition should be extra careful during seasonal changes.

4. Bad breath is one indication that your body has liver Qi stagnation. This condition can, in turn, cause your stomach Qi to overheat. Emotional problems or stress can bring on this kind of bad breath. Look for healthy ways to relieve any emotional discomfort especially if it is chronic. For instance, TCM has one way to reduce stress. As we've seen, you can buy a dozen eggs and smash them. Or, you can smash raw potatoes by stomping on them. Or, in a safe place, break glass bottles. Though these actions may seem a little unusual, they are time-tested TCM ways to help relieve anger. Fried, barbecued, and/or spicy foods can generate excess heat in your stomach and eventually cause a stomach function disorder. Try to avoid these foods whenever possible. Make sure you have regular bowel movements.

5. If you do not have a physical problem with your ears, ringing or tinnitus in the ears means you have a kidney Qi deficiency. You should regard this as a serious health sign because, according to TCM, the kidney is the foundation of the body's overall Qi. For women going through menopause, this is a particularly serious sign, because a kidney Qi deficiency is one of the two major causes of menopausal symptoms. There are certain foods you can add to your diet to help increase kidney Qi. Eat any kind of seafood, including shrimp, lobster, clams, oysters, salmon, tuna, etc. You can also add black beans, roasted walnuts, and other nuts as often as possible. When this condition persists, TCM treats it with herbs and acupuncture.

6. TCM believes that you can identify internal health conditions by examining of external physical signs. For instance, your nails are the mirrors of your liver. If your liver is healthy, your nails should be shiny, grow fast, and not break easily. If your nails are in poor condition and crack or break easily, your liver function is out of balance and you must treat it. Gelatin, shellfish, and clams can help your nails improve. Examine your nails periodically, if the half moons are not white and full, your liver Qi is weakening or becoming deficient. Take care of yourself, this is an early warning sign of internal imbalances.

7. In TCM theory, if the nose area is red, then the stomach is suffering from excess heat. This condition is also sometimes related to unbalanced liver function. Unless the condition is fixed from the inside out, most treatments are temporary. Acupuncture, herbs, and lifestyle changes can help alleviate this condition.

8. The eyes are the "window" of the liver. If your eyes tear frequently, or if you wake up with matter in your eyes, your liver Qi is stagnating. A liver Qi dysfunction has now progressed to a physical problem. It is important to treat the root cause of this condition before it progresses further and reaches more advanced stages. Acupuncture, herbs, and lifestyle changes can also make a beneficial difference.

9. According to TCM theory, the meridians of six different organs run through the head. Qi stagnation in one or a combination of these meridians can theoretically cause 720 different kinds of headaches ($6 \times 5 \times 4 \times 3 \times 2 \times 1 = 720$). To treat a headache effectively, it is essential to identify which organ is out of balance. For instance, headaches on either side of the head relate to the gallbladder; headaches at the front of the head relate to the stom-

ach; and headaches at the top of the head are associated with the liver and kidney.

Taking painkillers may alleviate headaches temporarily, but they can mask more serious problems that can emerge later. As you can see, headaches are merely symptoms telling you that there is a deeper problem, which resides in one or more of your five major organs. You can also see that headaches are specific to the individual. Your husband's headache may be different from yours, as yours may be different from your mother's. That is why pain relievers only work for some people some of the time.

10. If you have adult acne, TCM theory states that your liver and kidney organs are out of balance and not functioning in harmony. The messages that they need to exchange to keep your skin clear and unblemished are not being communicated properly. Unless you restore balance in this important relationship, it is unlikely that your acne will improve permanently with topical treatments. TCM believes that it is essential to treat adult acne from the inside out. Chronic anger and stress are two of the major causes of this condition.

Follow yin/yang's law and there is life.
Go against yin/yang's law and there is death.
Following yin/yang's law, disease can be cured,
Going against yin/yang's law, disease can become
uncontrollable

Therefore, the wise man does not fix the disease at
hand,
but treats tomorrow's.
Therefore, the wise man doesn't rein in the chaos of the
moment,
but tames tomorrow's.

NEI JING (475-221 B.C.)

CHAPTER 12

THE SECRET OF SUCCESSFUL SELF-HEALING FOR WOMEN IN TRANSITION:
How to Help Your Body, Mind, and Spirit Work as One

THE understanding of Qi is the true foundation of TCM. It governs its principles and its theories. The tools and techniques we've discussed are merely conveyances of Qi, or healing energy, between the doctor and the patient.

The deeper his or her understanding of Qi, the more powerful and effective the treatment. The best doctors really heal by Qi, and need to use only a few techniques, herbs, or acupuncture needles. If they are extraordinary, maybe all he or she needs to do is simply talk with you. That is the highest level of TCM practice, because there is no intermediary. If your Qi and your doctor's can really connect, you should consider yourself very fortunate. The ancients described this as "two stars that collide with each other. The power of both ignites as one." Given the high-tech medical environment of today, many people may find this form of medicine difficult to comprehend. It is, however, true and this ancient medical system has been practiced this way for far more than five thousand years. But for it to work, you must be open to the experience.

Remember that even the best doctor can only fix the fixable problems. He or she cannot save your life. No one can save your life but you. Your life is in your own hands, and heaven's. TCM has a saying, "Your life belongs to heaven; your health belongs to you." That is why it is essential for you to take responsibility for your own healing. Never is this more critical for women than during menopause. As I have said, this is the last great opportunity to become really healthy for the rest of your life.

TCM's specialty is prevention. I hope that you've learned a great deal about the value of prevention in this book. If you can keep yourself from becoming unbalanced in the first place, you can avoid a tremendous range of activities and pathogens, both internal and external, that can ultimately affect the quality and quantity of your life. You can live that much longer to develop and enrich your body, mind, and spirit. You will have that much more time to deepen your connections with Universal Qi and its true, unconditional love for all things and all people. You will have the opportunity to expand your spiritual dimensions and touch that which is eternal within you.

KEEPING A PEACEFUL HEART

If you are serious about taking advantage of life's last great opportunity to heal yourself, you now know that you must make the necessary shifts in the way you manage your daily life. If you want to strengthen yourself so that your body continues to produce enough estrogen for the rest of your life, you can start right now by applying the wisdom of TCM. If you really want to avoid ERT or HRT and eliminate the hot flashes, night sweats, heart palpitations, headaches, mood swings, digestive problems, and other discomforts of menopause, then begin by letting this self-healing process permeate everything you do. It's not a chore to accomplish, but a joyful, healthful way of living every day in the present.

This process begins with your heart, the king who controls the energy activity of your whole body: physical, mental, emotional, and spiritual. The heart is the master message center for all your organs, and so the state of your heart has a profound effect on the whole realm of the body and mind. If the king is upset, he will pass along his unhappiness to all the other organs. Then everyone will be upset. This is not a mental concept. This is a physiological process understood for millennia that I want to share with you. On the other hand, a peaceful heart can help all the other organs function well, especially your liver.

One of the main goals, then, in self-healing is to make the king more peaceful. Your heart must be in the right place, and the right place is what TCM terms a "baby place": peaceful, loving, and clear. When I tell this to my Western women patients, they understand what I mean, but look dismayed at what appears to be an enormous task of trying to achieve this state, given the lifestyles they're living. I tell them that it is not as hard as it sounds.

As we know so well, women today, especially in Western societies, live with tremendous stress. They seem to have an endless round of responsibilities that not only includes their work and family, but extended families, aging and ill parents, volunteer tasks and relentless demands for their time and attention. It's no wonder that women find the idea of making any part of their lives peaceful such a big task. There is so much in their daily lives that conspires against a peaceful heart. Menopause, which is a major cyclical turning point for the body and its Qi, puts even more pressure on the heart, because its relationship with the kidney is not as strong as it was in younger days.

It is crucial to do your best to reduce stress in your life and to control your emotions. Stress is not just mental concept. It is a physical danger to you and a very real threat to your organs and your health. Tell yourself that stress is a very real enemy—and believe it! This involves a lot of letting go: keeping life as simple as you can, not being too angry or fearful, not worrying or thinking too much. It also involves having a constant awareness of the kind of messages you are sending yourself, and trying to make them as positive as possible. Remember that the power of your mental Qi or energy to help or hinder change is very strong. If you trust and believe in yourself and always give yourself a positive message of

"I can do it; I can become stronger; I can heal myself," you will lend tremendous support to the healing process.

Negativity and doubt have the opposite effect, and can do a lot to undermine your best efforts to change. Constantly remind yourself to take care of yourself. This can take the form of hanging up a special picture that makes you feel calm and happy in a room where you spend a lot of time, listening to your favorite music, or keeping fresh flowers on your desk, or in your home. There are many things outside you that cannot be changed, but you do have the power to create your own peace and balance within. Chaos may reign around you, but if you've developed inner strength, you don't have to let it knock you off center.

This means taking responsibility. Don't blame others for your stress, or let anything get in the way of your forward momentum of healing and change. If your own Qi is strong and balanced, negative energy from the outside cannot infect you. The key point is keeping yourself peaceful. In this stressful world, many women think they should be doing even more to "get on top of" their lives. Sometimes, they may feel unlucky because, from the outside it appears that so many things are happening to them. Here's an ancient story that might help you learn how to look a different way at the things that happen to you and how to recognize fortune in "misfortune."

LUCKY AND UNLUCKY

In a small ancient Chinese village, a mother had three daughters, and one son. She complained constantly that she was unlucky. It seemed that everything that could befall a woman, had happened to her. She worked from morning until night. Her house was tiny and always needed fixing. Her daughters were unmarried. They never had enough food. Often, they relied on the son to find work to make ends meet. She complained day and night to the gods that she was indeed an unlucky woman.

Winter was very hard for the whole family. In the spring,

her only son went to a neighboring village to buy some grain. On his return, he fell off his horse and broke his leg. His much-needed help in planting the spring crop would be minimal. As he returned to his mother, she was beside herself. Again, she told the gods how sad she was and how badly she thought fate was treating her. Shortly thereafter, the prince who ruled her region sent a large army to look for young men who were fit to fight in his next battle. Seeing the condition of the woman's son, they passed him by saying he could never serve in battle. From that day forward, the woman considered herself a very lucky woman.

Who then is lucky? It depends on whose point of view it is and the point in time they decide on what is lucky. In this case, the mother and the son are both lucky. The son is lucky because he was saved from almost certain death in battle. The mother is lucky because her male child remains with her to pass along the culture of the family. In the same way today, things happen that appear unlucky at the time, but may turn out to be very lucky in the end.

A few people have the experience of having their car break down, or of having some other event, interfere with their ability to make an airplane flight. The plane crashes, but the person avoids that catastrophe because of luck. It is human nature to judge the events in front of us as indicative of the way our life is going, but if you want to keep a peaceful heart, it's important to remember that events are not necessarily what they seem. For instance, many of us pursue dreams of winning the lottery, even just a small windfall of money, we believe, will change our lives for the better. And, for some people it will. However, a survey of people who have won the lottery tells us that most are unhappy with what their lives have become after winning. Who then is lucky?

When things happen in your life, learn to look at them with a peaceful heart. You will have come a long way in helping to keep your body, mind, and spirit in good health.

FENG SHUI

Feng Shui (FUNG SCHWAY) is one tool you can use to become healthier and more peaceful. In ancient times, if you were sick, you would first go to a doctor, then to a Feng Shui master. Feng Shui is actually also a kind of energy treatment. TCM believes that illness is an indication that we've become disconnected from the balanced Qi of the Universe. The true healing purpose of Feng Shui then is to find a way to reconnect the individual's Qi with that of the Universe's.

Feng means "wind." Wind is a power that belongs to heaven, and it can carry many different kinds of Qi or energy. Shui means "water." Water can also carry Qi and it has the ability to flow everywhere. Its power belongs to earth. Wind and water represent the two elements in our lives: our fate, which we cannot change (heaven); and the aspects of our lives that we can change (earth).

Feng Shui is always used for a specific purpose. For instance, you can set up your home or workplace to improve your health, to bring luck, or to make more money. It is not an all-purpose practice. A Feng Shui master should always ask you what you want to achieve. Again, TCM is a healing system that relates all things to the individual and her needs. Remember that what works for a friend or colleague in their home or office may not work for you. Your Feng Shui configuration of space and materials must be based on you and your own unique Qi. To be truly effective, it must be based on the ancient treatment principles of TCM, which looks at: who you are, how you are, when you are, and where you are. While it is not possible to provide a "one size fits all" description of how to use Feng Shui, here are some general principles that you can use to create a more balanced and harmonious environment:

- A place that is light, open, and quiet is best. If you always feel vaguely uncomfortable in a particular area, you're unconsciously reacting to the Qi of this space or place: This space may be too small, too dark, closed in, or too noisy. You want the feeling to be smooth and flowing, definitely not crowded or busy. Try to make your work space reflect these qualities to the best of your ability. Above all, strive to make your home this way.

- One easy method of creating a smooth, flowing feeling is to eliminate sharp edges. The most harmonious shape is the circle: it is the shape of the structures of our bodies, and the whole universe. Try to eliminate the harsh edges and the sharp angles in your environment and revise what you can.

- Feng Shui works best when it makes use of living things. Plants, for example, have a lot of healing power. Remember our discussion of Qi in Chapter 3? Everything communicates through Qi. Plants do have the ability to communicate with you through Qi and support and strengthen your own Qi in the process. Since plants are especially good for healing liver dysfunctions, they can help women going through menopause feel better. Surround yourself at work and at home with easy-to-care-for plants or fresh flowers. Remember that TCM considers the liver to be the most important organ for women's health. If you tend to feel angry or depressed frequently, plants and flowers can really help you feel more peaceful. They represent a minor investment for a major benefit!

- You can also use the Five Element Theory to support the Qi of particular organs. For instance, anything with a green or deep blue (colors that match the liver's own Qi) will help your liver. If you work on a computer, keep a plant or something green nearby. This will help offset the drain on your liver Qi caused by long hours of looking into the screen (as will stopping to close your eyes for awhile every couple of hours). Another way to help relieve eyestrain is to gently massage the canthus or the small ball at the inside of your eye. Why? Because the eyes are the opening gate to the outside world of the liver. Too much looking can actually damage liver function.

- Excessive heat is also bad for the liver, so if you tend to be angry or to have other problems related to the liver, it's important to try and remain calm. The kidney, on the other hand, is harmed by excessive cold. Keep these simple facts in mind when the indoor or outdoor climates you're exposed to become excessive. Become conscious that you want to stay in a balanced state. If it's too hot in a room you're in, change the temperature, if possible, or move to a cooler spot. If it's too hot outdoors, cool yourself off and don't overexert yourself. Likewise, if it's too cold—inside or out—seek warmth. If it's not possible for you to go south for the winter, at least do your best to stay warm.

THE SECRET OF INCREASING QI

A big part of increasing your Qi for healing in your daily life is learning how to conserve it in the first place. It isn't enough just to build it up—if you then waste Qi or allow it to drain away, your efforts are in vain. This becomes increasingly important as you progress through the seven-year energy cycles we discussed. It is particularly important when you start to move through the sixth and seventh cycles and enter menopause. Younger women need to think far ahead (I'll admit that's not the way in our Western society and probably difficult to do for many). Menopausal or postmenopausal women need to be more careful and more conscious about managing Qi than they were when they were younger.

A good way to begin to conserve your Qi is to recognize the value of slowing down. We end up losing a lot of Qi if our lives are very complicated, and move too fast. Try to take it easy. If you can slow down the use of your Qi, you will slow its decline as well. There is a very real benefit in doing this; you can live a longer healthier life. Just stop for a minute and think of the things that are important to you. Now, think about being able to enjoy them as a vibrant healthy older woman alive with enthusiasm, energy, and spirit.

Try to do nothing more often. For instance, be aware of how you begin your day. If you work in an office, instead of immediately checking your e-mail and your telephone messages, sit down and close your eyes, even if only for a few minutes. You just need to get into the habit of separating your body, mind, and spirit from the frenetic pace surrounding you. This is something you can also do any time during the day when things get hectic, or out of control. If you feel yourself becoming tense and harried, stop what you're doing, and just sit quietly for a few minutes. Close your eyes, and breathe slowly and deeply from your diaphragm. To help you calm down, reverse your natural way of breathing so that your abdomen flattens when you inhale, and pushes out when you exhale.

Tension consumes a lot of Qi. If you relax, and become more peaceful both internally and externally, you can save your Qi instead of spending it. Imagine, just by resting or staying relaxed, you can bank healing Qi for when you really need it. Incorporating these seemingly small steps into your everyday life can make a big difference. I tell my patients, "It can even change your life completely." Until they try it for themselves, they have been trained to believe that something so simple and so truthful can't be effective. Here's an example: If every time you get in your car, you take just a few minutes to sit quietly and make sure you are calm before you start driving, you might avoid an accident that could easily have happened had you rushed off.

When I first talk with women about these things, they say something like, "You don't understand. I have a really busy life. I can't see anything I could stop or cut out. You don't understand. What I really need is a few more hours in the day to get everything done. I have a lot of responsibility. I have to keep moving or everything will fall apart!" I feel so sorry for these women. They have convinced themselves that the things they do are more important than their own health and, in effect, their own life. Of course, there is very little in our Western culture that supports their slowing down either. All of us have been conditioned to "be productive," even at the expense of our own health. I tell my patients this is not right. So, until we meet, all their internal and external messages are the same: "You're only valuable as long as you can keep driving yourself."

But, Western society has a saying that "Everyone is replaceable." So, don't think that you are the only person who can do what you can do. I suggest to them, as I do to you, that you can change your internal tape and you can play a new one! The only thing that's not replaceable is your own health. Many times, women tell me: "Oh, I would feel useless (or lazy) if I didn't do what I'm doing." Yet, they're basically killing themselves with their lifestyle choices. Here's a story that illustrates the true meaning of useless and useful. I hope you will take some time out to consider what is really useful in your life.

USELESS AND USEFUL

One day, a master and his student were out gathering wood to build a house. As they went up and down the mountain, the student would run to one tree and then another and ask his master, "How about this one? Isn't this a good one to cut down?" The young student's master would nod yes to this tree, and sometimes no to that tree.

Now, most of these trees were in their prime; they had not yet grown very old and were immediately cut down for building material. One day, the student was out with his master and they came upon a very large tree that had obviously lived a long and healthy life. "Master, this must be one of the best trees of all, don't you think?" he said. "No," replied the master, "this tree is not useful for us. It is not useful for home-building because it is the kind of tree that harbors termites. It isn't very good for building boats, because it is not light enough to float easily. We can't make a wooden jar out of it to hold water and wine, because it is too porous and the liquid will leak out of it. This kind of tree is useless to us." The student thought for a while, then said, "Master, I don't understand—because the tree is useless, it can stand here forever, and that is useful, at least to the tree. So, is the tree useless or useful? The master replied, "Useful and useless are a matter of who is looking and from what point of view they are looking. For us, this tree is useless because it offers nothing. For the tree, its usefulness lies in its uselessness because that is what has saved its life. All the useful trees have already been cut down for houses and coffins; their usefulness has ended their lives early."

One of the most important principles of conserving Qi is moderation. Don't overdo anything. This applies not only to physical activities such as work, exercise, and sex, but to mental activities as well. When you overuse your mind, you lose even more Qi than you do when you overexert yourself physically. Thinking too much, worrying too much, even loving too much, all take a toll on your precious Qi, or life force.

Learning to conserve Qi means learning how to save more than you spend. A woman in menopause needs as much Qi as possible to counteract her body's natural kidney Qi decline. First, you must develop an awareness of all the ways that you waste Qi, and then make a concerted and systematic effort to eliminate them. Think about it like this: if you pour water into a pitcher full of holes, it will never fill up. If you want to have a full pitcher of water, you must first fix the leaks. In the case of Qi, when you do this, all of your efforts to both generate and conserve it will make a difference and add up to a tremendous change.

FINDING THE RIGHT EXERCISE AND GETTING THE MOST OUT OF IT

Getting the right kind of exercise is also very important to building up your Qi. Most people recognize the importance of exercise in maintaining health, but they may not understand that different kinds of exercise differ widely in their effect. Many popular forms of exercise, for instance jogging and intensive aerobics, actually waste more Qi than they help you generate. If you go out running in the wind, rain, or cold, you expend even more Qi as your body battles with these natural forces to stay balanced and fend off external pathogens related to climate.

Because I practice in New York City, you can imagine the number of women I work with who are what today's society applauds as "hard chargers." They are absolutely shocked when I discuss exercise with them. Many have been pounding treadmills, or bouncing on trampolines for years. Eventually, when they come to understand the principles of TCM, we have a lot of fun talking about their old lifestyle. I joke with them and ask: "What are you doing? Do you want cow muscles? Or cat muscles?" You know how cats act. One minute they can be sleeping soundly and the next they are springing gracefully into the air to catch something. They can move in this beautiful fluid way because their tendons are flexible. Their muscles are lean. Cows, on the other hand, have huge muscles, but they will fall over and hurt themselves if they don't move right. Naturally, the answer is you want to have long, flexible tendons that will support your flexibility and range of motion well into your later years. I urge my patients and you to be careful where you expend your physical energy.

Also, you might be interested to know that, according to TCM theories, finishing off your physical routine with a big cold drink compounds the damage to your Qi. You shouldn't eat or drink for at least half an hour after exercising. Why? Because although your physical body has stopped moving, your internal Qi has not and is still circulating through your body. You have to give your Qi a chance to cool and calm down. Jogging and aerobics— especially step aerobics—are also bad for your knees and, more importantly, your tendons. Ultimately, this is not good for your tendons, which are the "tissue" of your liver, and can ultimately affect the healthy functioning of this organ. As I mentioned earlier, many of the women I see for chronic fatigue syndrome have a history of overexercising.

When you consider an exercise routine, think about the fact that our bodies are close to 70 percent water. If you approach this from the TCM perspective, you will understand that the best results can be gained by acting in harmony with the natural law. The kinds of exercise you choose should match the nature of your body. Exercises, especially for women going through menopause, should be energy-giving; they should also be water-like, soft and not hard. Some healthful forms of exercise are Qigong, Taiji, yoga, walking in nature (not on a treadmill), and noncompetitive swimming. Stretching—with a particular focus on lengthening and loosening the tendons—is also very good, and will help your liver which governs the state of these structures.

Developing softness and flexibility is much better for both your body and your Qi than simply building muscle. Weight training and other strenuous forms of exercise that create big hard muscles—like the "cow" muscles we just talked about—make you less flexible, more vulnerable to injury, and, in a sense, less strong. In China, the concept of strength is quite different than it is in the West. The goal of physical training is not to build up a muscle mass, but to increase flexibility, agility, and the kind of springlike power that comes from long, loose tendons. A body with hard, overdeveloped muscles can become dense and lumbering, and not flowing or elegant. The ideal, especially in martial arts forms, which originally were healing arts forms, is that of the cat—soft and swift. The next time you think about your exercise routine, study a cat. See how she seems to sleep her life away. Her body is relaxed and fluid. Yet when the need arises, she can move with speed, grace, and power.

Whatever physical routines you undertake, don't overdo it. Don't force your body to exercise too much. Many women tell me how great it feels, even when they're on the verge of fatigue, to go to their gyms and work out for an hour or more. They say, "Oh, it makes me really feel so much better. I just have to force myself to go. You know once I'm there, I can get into it and I feel like I have so much more energy!" I tell them, "Of course, you do. You've just been able to release a lot of stress from your body. However, the Qi that you spent to make this happen, you could have used a different way to gain the same benefits. If you don't have enough Qi from your digestive function, you are using up your kidney Qi. You might want to think about that, because it's the very thing you'll need as you grow older."

And, unless you want to become like a machine, I recommend that you try to avoid exercise machines. To get the most from exercise, you should use your body in a natural way. And when you are exercising your body, you should also be exercising your mind. How can a dead machine help you train your mind?

I recommend that all my patients take a walk instead, and practice being peaceful at the same time. Don't walk too fast or too far. You want to feel relaxed and calm after your walk; you don't want a pounding heart and a body bathed in sweat. If you live in the city, try to walk in a park, or someplace where you can connect with nature and enjoy natural sounds and a calm feeling as you exercise. (Yes, you are really exercising when you're walking mindfully in nature.) If you're rushing around plugged into a portable radio, you will miss the opportunity of tuning up your own body with nature's healing Qi, and the rhythms of the natural world around you. Listen to the birds, let your mind be peaceful, forget about who and where you are. You may find that the trees or the animals have something to tell you. They can all communicate through Qi. Why not you?

There are also many simple ways to "exercise" your Qi while you're standing or sitting or engaged in the regular activities of daily life. If you're feeling stressed, gently massage the inner canthus of your eyes, or your temples. You can also rub the sides of your head in an arc from your temples back over your ears. The gallbladder meridian runs through this area, so massaging this meridian is also good for its partner organ, your liver, as well as your skin and hair. The gallbladder and liver meridians also run along the sides of your rib cage, so you can rub this area too. And there are liver points under the breast in line with the nipple (find the spot that feels sensitive) that you can massage while you're taking a shower.

Another good stress release exercise is to take your hairbrush and, with the bristle side down, hit the outside and inside of your legs. My menopause patients love this one. Hit as hard as you can—it should even hurt a little. Always do this instant "energy massage" in a downward motion—not up and down. What are you doing? You're stimulating the six meridians that run through your leg—liver, spleen, kidney, gallbladder, stomach, and bladder—and the flow of their Qi. To help increase Qi, you can also rub your kidney and the two major points I've mentioned before, *Guanyuan* (four fingers below your navel) and *Mingmen* (at the small of your back at belt level). And for a quick overall tuneup, rub your ears vigorously with the palms of your hands until they're very warm. The ears, which are the opening of the kidney, are also a microcosm of the entire body. Many key acupoints are located on the ears and rubbing them frequently can stimulate your whole energy system. This offers a good "whole body" tuneup, especially for women entering their sixth and seventh energy cycles.

CHAPTER 13

WU MING MERIDIAN THERAPY:
Ancient Energy Movements and Postures You Can Perform Daily for Self-Healing

*T*HE most important part of our Seven-Point Guide to Self-Healing with TCM (in Chapter 2) is *Wu Ming* Meridian Therapy. I have developed these exclusive ancient energy movements with my master, Professor Xi-hua Xu of Yunnan, China. Professor Xu is a well-respected expert on the use of Qigong for medical purposes. He has worked at the highest levels of the Chinese government. One of his special gifts is the ability to understand meridians and meridian blockages from an energy or Qi standpoint, and the medical conditions to which they are related. We have spent many hours discussing Western women and menopause and why their many symptoms cause so much distress. We also talked about which movements could benefit Western women the most so that they can move through menopause and manage its symptoms without ERT or HRT. The result is this specially created Qigong practice for you.

Our *Wu Ming* Meridian Therapy is based on ancient meridian theory that we've already talked about previously. Remember, as we have emphasized throughout this book, when your organs function in harmony and Qi flows freely or unobstructed through your meridians, it is not possible for illness or disease to enter your body. This is the state that you want to move toward.

Understanding the importance of the "healing message" behind *Wu Ming* Meridian Therapy is like understanding the performance of a great musician. While this musician might be able to teach his or her best students techniques for making beautiful music, he or she can only pass along the spirit or soul of the performance. This part can't be taught, but it can be known.

In TCM, the best healing knowledge is passed similarly from master to student—often over the course of centuries and even millennia. Our system comes from such an ancient lineage. In a similar way, I am passing on to you a special "healing message" with our unique *Wu Ming* Meridian Therapy. Following my instructions for these movements will convey important healing benefits to you. Through continual practice, you will have many opportunities to receive the strong healing message behind this unique Qigong form. How can these seemingly simple movements make powerful changes in your body, mind, and spirit? Not only can your practice help your body's Qi come back into balance, but it can help you reach a new level of internal harmony where you can connect with and receive Universal Qi. Image how amazing it is to really have a channel or conduit to an endless sea of unconditional love and unlimited Qi, or life force. While the physical rewards are substantial, the spiritual gifts of *Wu Ming* Meridian Therapy can lead you to a place of great peace and beauty.

All of the following Qigong movements refer to the dragon. In Chinese culture the dragon actually represents the spirit of China itself. In TCM, the dragon represents the energy of the liver, which is most appropriate here since this ancient medical system regards the liver as the most important organ for women's health. I recommend that you practice the full set of eight self-healing movements daily. As your practice develops, you will gradually help unblock any stagnating Qi and begin to experience less menopausal discomforts. You can chart your progress in reducing these symptoms in the section of the TCM Self-Healing Evaluation Form that relates to frequency of symptoms. If you cannot practice every day, try your best to incorporate as many movements as possible into your daily routine. I work with many women going through menopause. They tell me that once they start practicing *Wu Ming* Meridian Therapy, it becomes the most important part of their day. Why? Because it makes them feel so well. Remember, this is your opportunity to take control of your own health and healing. The results can be remarkable. Here are some simple guidelines for getting the most out of your *Wu Ming* Meridian Therapy practice.

1. Always practice in comfortable clothing.

2. Try to practice at least once a day and at the same time. The entire program of eight movements should take twenty-five or thirty minutes a day. A good time to increase Qi is from 11:00 A.M. to 1:00 P.M. and from 5:00 P.M. to 7:00 P.M. It's also good to practice during the full moon, as well as during seasonal transitions like the winter solstice, spring equinox, and so on. Your birthday and birth time and your parents' birthdays are also especially good times to practice.

3. Practice each movement individually whenever you can. Besides practicing the entire set together, I recommend you try to find time during your day to work in each movement individually. For maximum benefit, you must practice a specific movement for at least five minutes, when you perform them separately. The last movement is designed to build harmony among all your organs and help strengthen kidney Qi. Try to hold this posture for as long as possible; the longer the better. If you practice long enough, you can help your body, mind, and spirit become one.

4. Breathe naturally. *Wu Ming* Meridian Therapy requires no special breathing techniques.

5. Let your mind go. In *Wu Ming* Meridian Therapy there is no special mental focus. Try to remain peaceful and concentrate on what you are doing. Before practice try some slow deep breathing and give yourself an overall positive message of self-healing. Do not focus on a particular organ or meridian. If your mind cannot remain peaceful, then try to focus on the thought that you are receiving natural healing Qi from the sun, the moon, the stars, the entire Universe. At the same time, imagine that this natural healing Qi is filling your body and rebalancing your organs so that they can work in harmony as they were always meant to do. See yourself becoming healthier and healthier.

6. Accept and believe in your natural healing ability. When you reach a certain level in this particular ancient self-healing Qigong system, you will notice that the Qigong energy itself will cut off your thoughts and help you enter a timeless space where you can access your own self-healing power.

7. Do not practice when you are very hungry, after a big meal, if you are very tired, or after sex.

8. Do each movement slowly. These are not aerobic or physical exercises. They are very gentle meridian stretches.

THE DRAGON PULLS ITS TAIL FROM THE SEA

1. Stand with your feet parallel, shoulder-width apart.
2. Make a fist with your right hand, with your index finger pointing straight down, and your palm facing backward. Do this movement slowly and make sure your finger feels very heavy like it is pulling something from below.

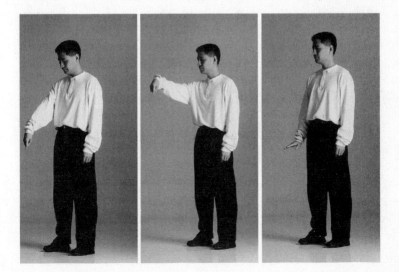

3. Slowly pull your hand up to shoulder height.
4. Open your hand, and let your arm slowly drop to your side.
5. Repeat the same movement with your left hand.
6. Repeat these movements for three to five minutes.

WAKING THE DRAGON'S ENERGY

1. Stand with your feet parallel, shoulder-width apart.
2. Raise your hands in front of your body, then let them drop down and back so that your palms hit your abdomen below the navel between your hip bones. Your wrists should be relaxed, and you should hit very softly.
3. Continue this movement for three to five minutes.

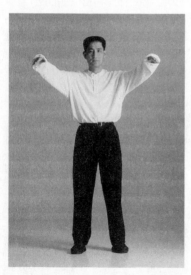 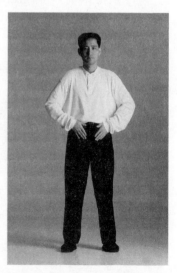

THE DRAGON JUMPS INTO THE SEA

1. Stand with your feet together. Place your hands palm up touching the sides of your waist, and make a fist, with your index finger pointing forward.

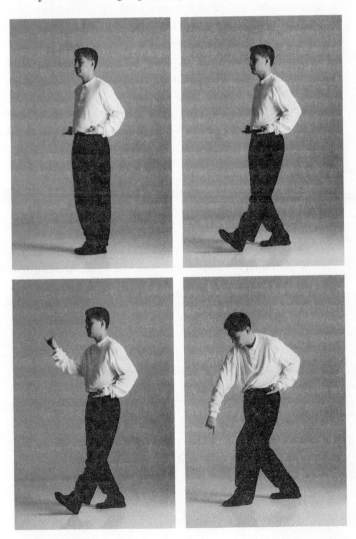

2. Step forward with your left foot, and touch it to the floor with your heel down. Your weight should remain on the back of your leg.

3. Raise your right fist with the index finger extended until it's in front of your shoulder.

4. Turn your extended arm counterclockwise until your index finger ends up facing down and your palm faces outward. Make sure your palm does not face backward. Shift your weight forward as you push your finger toward the floor.

5. Shift your weight back to the Step 2 position.

6. Then return to the Step 1 position.

7. Repeat the same movements on the opposite side, with your right foot and left hand. Both movements count as one. Be sure you do this very slowly.

8. Continue this movement for three to five minutes.

THE DRAGON'S TOE DANCE

1. Stand with your feet parallel, shoulder-width apart. Put your hands on your waist, and shift your weight to your

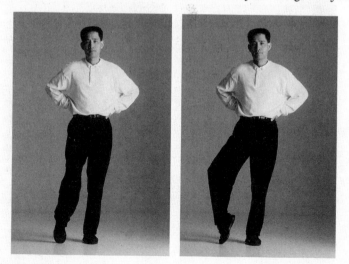

left side. Raise your right heel, keeping your toe on the floor.

2. Slowly make a circle outward with your whole leg, keeping your toe on the floor. Make sure your ankle, knee, and hip joints turn together at the same time. Each circle counts as one. Count three sets of eight.

3. Shift your weight to your right side, slowly raise your left heel, and repeat the same circling movement with your right leg. Count three sets of eight.

THE DRAGON'S STRETCH

1. Stand with your feet parallel, shoulder-width apart.

2. Squat down as low as you can without bringing your heels off the floor, stretch your arms out in front of you, and place your palms flat on the floor.

3. Keep your palms on the floor while you straighten your legs up as high as you can. Continue very slowly to move

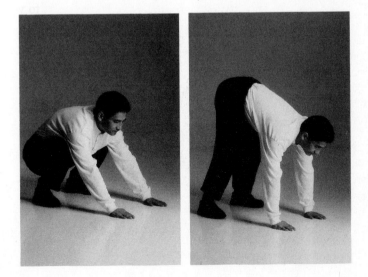

down and up with your palms and feet on the floor. Think about how a cat stretches.

4. Repeat for three to five minutes.

THE DRAGON KICKS BACKWARD

1. Stand with your feet parallel, shoulder-width apart, and put your hands on your waist.
2. Bend your left knee, then kick straight back with your heel. Make sure your leg is stretched out, and that you do not kick too high.
3. Each kick backward counts as one.
4. Do the same with your right leg.
5. Count eight times twice for each leg. If you feel a bit wobbly, this is an indication that your physical strength is weak. Hold onto a chair or table edge lightly. As your practice progresses, you will get stronger and this should eventually disappear.

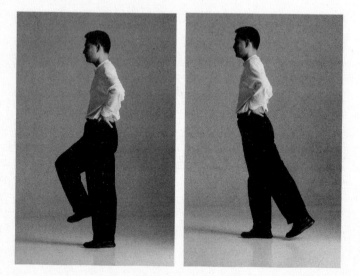

THE DRAGON CIRCLES WITH THE MOON

1. Lie on your back on a rug or exercise mat. Bring your knees up to your chest, and hold them there so that your body remains in a curled-up position. Keep your neck and upper back off the floor.
2. Center your weight over your back. Use your stomach muscles to help you rock your body from left to right, shifting your position slightly each time so that you turn in a small circle. Go slowly, and try to use your whole body.
3. After each circle reverse direction. For the sake of balance, circle to the left and right an equal amount of times. This movement can really strengthen your kidney Qi. The more you practice, the more benefit you will receive.
4. Make a circle clockwise first; then reverse the direction.
5. Do this entire movement for about two minutes.

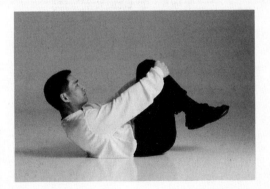

HOLDING THE DRAGON'S BALL

1. Stand with your feet parallel, shoulder-width apart; bend your knees slightly.
2. Bring your hands up comfortably and naturally so that your palms are in front of your navel area, as if you were holding a ball of energy.

3. Close your eyes. Try to stand in this position for at least five minutes. The longer you can hold this ancient Qigong position, the more healing benefits you will gain.

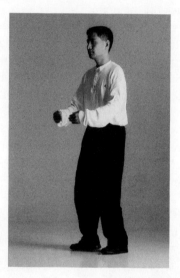

CHAPTER 14

SECRET ENERGY GATES THAT CAN HELP YOU GO THROUGH MENOPAUSE SUCCESSFULLY

*I*N the human body, there are many special acupoints or "energy gates" that can help your organs communicate with each other harmoniously. Like the junction where several major highways come together, these points let a maximum amount of Qi or energy flow through. Some points are stronger than others and can help you accumulate more healing Qi. How to locate some of these points and apply their healing benefits for specific problems is knowledge that is not necessarily found in TCM medical texts. Rather, it's information passed along for many generations from master to student. I have been fortunate enough to receive this kind of high-level medical knowledge from several of my masters. It is my privilege to share this gift with you.

Massaging these points can help you reduce a range of symptoms TCM considers early warning signals of critical imbalances and Qi or energy dysfunctions. Incorporating acupressure into your daily routine, can help your organs function in harmony. When you accomplish this, you can gain more strength and more Qi to manage your menopausal symptoms.

Most of these healing gates are bilateral or located on each side of your body. You can massage individual points or a combination. I recommend that you massage each one for at least five

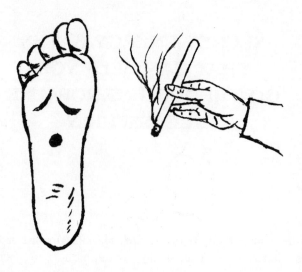

minutes a day for maximum effect. Here are special energy gates that you can work with:

1. This first important healing gate can help your body generate Qi to combat menopausal symptoms. It is also helpful in fighting breast cancer or preventing it. The point is located at the center of the bottom of each of your feet. You can massage this point with your thumb, or a tennis ball, or whatever you have on hand that helps stimulate it. This point can strengthen your whole body's Qi foundation. You can also use moxibustion to warm this point: cut a thin slice of fresh ginger about the size of a quarter, place it over this point, and use the heat of moxibustion to penetrate the ginger and drive its essence into this point. (Smokeless moxibustion sticks of herbs can be found at most Chinese herb stores, acupuncture medical supply companies, and Western natural food stores.) Do this for about five minutes on the bottom of each foot.

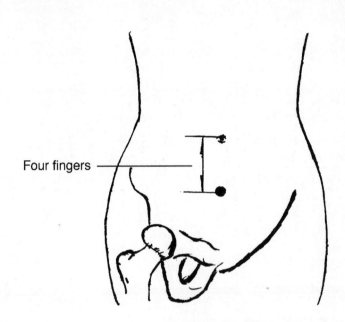

Four fingers

2. The second most important healing gate is located about the width of four fingers directly below your belly button. This point can also generate extra Qi for healing purposes and longevity. Massage this point gently in small circles in both directions. This point can help relieve menstrual cramps; help infertility; rebalance any kind of hormone problems, and help alleviate hot flashes, night sweats and vaginal discharge.

If you have breast or other kinds of cancer, or are undergoing chemotherapy or radiation, use ginger and moxibustion in the same way described above. In my opinion, from the energy point of view, this is one spot that is dangerous to stimulate with an acupuncture needle, especially during menopause.

3. From under your breastbone or sternum to above your belly button, there is an area that you can massage gently to generate more Qi for healing. Put one hand on top of the other with your palms on this area. Slowly and gently make a circle clockwise five times; reverse direction and make a circle counterclock-

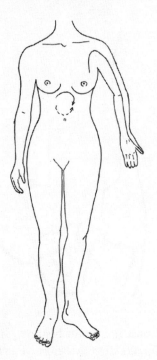

wise five times. Continue this routine for about five minutes. This can help strengthen your whole digestive system. It can also help relieve nausea and lack of appetite from chemotherapy.

4. There is a point that TCM refers to as *Mingmen* on your spine at the small of your back about where a belt would come. You can stimulate this point by hitting it gently with your fists in a swinging motion as you alternate each arm behind your back. This movement can help stimulate your kidney Qi. TCM considers this point your "life gate." Stimulating this point with an acupuncture needle can cause side effects. This is another point where I do not recommend letting anyone put an acupuncture needle.

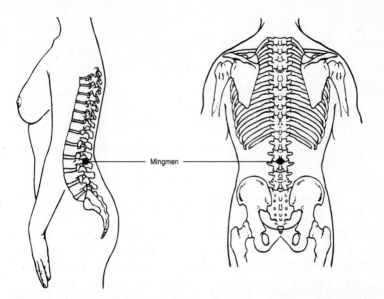

Mingmen

5. Where the two bones of the thumb and the index finger meet, there is another healing gate. It is located at the bottom of the index finger bone in the "V" shape. Using your opposite thumb, press or massage this point in a circle. After massaging this point, continue to gently massage the entire index finger bone toward the first knuckle of the index finger. This is a technique you can practice anywhere, anytime. This helps stimulate the Qi of the stomach, large intestine, and lung so that they begin to work in harmony, as they are supposed to do. If you find any soreness or tenderness in this area, massage it more deeply to unblock Qi stagnation.

6. Likewise, on the top of the foot, there is another healing gate where the big toe bone meets the second toe bone. Massage and press this spot with your thumb. Again, using your thumb, slide your finger continuously toward the tip of your second toe. You may feel some pain or discomfort; this means you are on the right spot and unblocking Qi stagnation in your liver meridian. This is a very important healing gate. (Remember the liver's im-

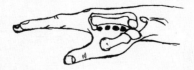

portance for women's health.) The degree of pain you feel will tell you how badly affected your liver function is. The more stressed you are, the more pain you will have. Try to massage this area frequently to keep liver Qi running smoothly.

7. There is a very easy way to stimulate a major energy gate that is better than any physical exercise you can do. It is so simple that you can do it anywhere at any time, and it requires no special clothing or equipment. I encourage you to do this as often as possible. When you are standing, just bend your knee very slightly and stamp your foot straight down lightly. Basically, this is like a marching step, only you should do it slowly and in a relaxed manner. The real trick is to keep your feet as flat as possible when you stamp them on the ground. The vibrations of this movement can actually waken and stimulate the Qi in all your meridians. The benefits are tremendous. Although it sounds almost too simple, I challenge you to do this Qigong movement and see how powerful the results are. Again, practice this movement for at least five minutes.

Stand before it and there is no beginning.
Follow it and there is no end.
Stay with the ancient Tao,
Move with the present.

TAO TE CHING (500-200 B.C.)

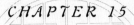

CHAPTER 15

HEALING FOODS AND RECIPES THAT HEAL:
Classical Herbs for Menopause

TCM believes that every food has a unique healing energy that can enter a particular organ(s) and its meridian. "Energy" in this sense means the essence or Qi of a food, not its caloric, nutritional, or chemical values. The healing Qi of all of the foods in the following list and recipes can support your kidney and liver, and the function of your digestive system. If you can revamp your eating habits to include these foods, TCM believes you will have much more control over your menopause and its symptoms. TCM also understands that you will be helping yourself go through this transition smoothly so that you can create an adequate amount of hormones for the rest of your life. Certain foods and herbs offer tremendous healing properties. I hope you will not underestimate their ability to make a major contribution to your self-healing work Let's look at these.

- *Seafood*: All seafood is very good for the kidney, especially shrimp, lobster, clams, oysters, salmon, tuna, etc. (remember that the flavor associated with the kidney is salty). If you like them, catfish and eel are also very good.
- *Nuts and Seeds*: Walnuts, pine nuts, and black sesame seeds are especially good for strengthening kidney Qi.

- *Beans*: Black and red beans are the best. Soybeans are good, but be careful not to eat too much tofu. Tofu has a cold essence or nature. Remember the stomach does not tolerate cold energy well.
- *Vegetables*: All deep green vegetables are good for supporting liver function (whose corresponding color is green), particularly broccoli and spinach. Mushrooms and scallions also help strengthen liver Qi. While Western nutrition focuses on their physical properties, TCM recognizes that behind this quality, the real reason they can help heal certain conditions is their property of Qi.
- *Cooking Oils*: Walnut and sesame oils are the best for the kidney.
- *Condiments*: Some condiments that are good for the digestive system are garlic, ginger, fennel, cinnamon, parsley, clove, and soy sauce.
- *Meat*: Try to avoid eating meat. Meat requires your body to expend extra Qi to digest it, and tends to have more toxins, antibiotics, and hormones than other kinds of food. If you do eat meat, lamb is the best. Pork is also good, as is free-range chicken, or the kind Chinese call black-bone chicken. The hormones in commercially raised, mass-produced chicken are not good, especially for young girls and women.

The following recipes are particularly healthful and can be used by women in either perimenopause or menopause. These healing foods can help support the function of your key organs. Try to incorporate them into your diet as much as possible. You may be surprised at how much changing your diet to these healing foods can help alleviate menopausal symptoms.

Baked Marinated Salmon with Scallions

This recipe is a delicious (and easy) way to combine two kidney-
and liver-nourishing foods. Use whole salmon, salmon fillets, or
steaks. Preheat the oven to 425° and then bake the fish with this
rule in mind: For each inch of thickness of the fish (measuring at
its thickest part), bake it for 10 minutes.

> *Oil for baking (such as corn)*
> *4 or 5 scallions*
> *Marinade (see below)*
> *Salmon, marinated overnight*

1. Cover the bottom of the baking dish with the oil (for an 8-inch
   by 12-inch baking dish, use about 6 tablespoons of oil).
2. Wash and trim the scallions, then cut them in half, lengthwise.
3. Line the oiled dish with the cut scallions, arranging them
   evenly over its surface.
4. Spoon half of the marinade (about 2½ tablespoons) over the
   scallions.
5. Place the salmon in the center of the dish on the bed of
   scallions.
6. Spoon the remaining marinade over the top of the fish.
7. Cover the dish with foil and refrigerate, allowing the fish to
   marinate overnight.
8. Remove dish from refrigerator and bake uncovered at 425°
   until fish is done.
9. Remove fish and scallions from dish and serve hot.

The Marinade

This recipe makes about 5 to 6 tablespoons of marinade, which is
enough for approximately 1 pound of fish. The ingredients can be
obtained at your local Chinese food store.

> *2 tablespoons Hoisin sauce*
> *1 tablespoon oyster sauce*
> *½ teaspoon fish sauce (or fish gravy)*

    2 teaspoons, finely chopped fresh ginger
    2 tablespoons mushroom-flavored soy sauce

Combine all ingredients thoroughly in a small-sized mixing bowl.

Mixed Vegetables

    Broccoli, cauliflower, and other vegetables of your choice
    Garlic cloves
    Fresh ginger root
    Sesame or walnut oil
    Soy sauce
    Black sesame seeds

Vegetable Medley

Cut vegetables into the sizes you like. Smash one or two garlic cloves. Peel skin off the fresh ginger and cut crosswise into ⅛ inch or thinner slices. Use about ½ of the ginger root. Put water into a pot large enough to hold all the vegetables. When the water boils, put in the garlic, ginger, and vegetables along with a few drops of sesame or walnut oil. Cook for 2 minutes or less, and drain vegetables.

SAUTÉED VEGETABLES

Put 1 teaspoon of sesame or walnut oil in a wok. Add one smashed garlic clove and sliced ginger to warm oil. Add vegetables and stir. Cook until vegetables are tender, but crisp. Do not overcook. Arrange vegetables on a platter and sprinkle with black sesame seeds.

STIR-FRIED VEGETABLES

Put 1 tablespoon of sesame oil in a wok. Heat oil until very hot (almost smoking). Add garlic and sliced ginger to taste. Add vegetables of your choice, and stir-fry until vegetables are crisp but tender. Again, do not overcook. Add soy sauce, and stir. Remove from heat. Arrange vegetables on a plate and sprinkle with black sesame seeds.

Vegetable Soup I

> *Plum tomatoes*
> *Zucchini*
> *Cauliflower*
> *Scallions*
> *Garlic*
> *Ginger*
> *Salt and pepper*
> *Sesame or walnut oil*

Sauté scallions, garlic, and ginger in a small amount of sesame or walnut oil. Add two diced plum tomatoes, stir, and add approximately 4 cups water. Add sliced zucchini and cauliflower. Add parsley if you like. Add salt and pepper to taste. Simmer until vegetables are of desired texture and soup is flavorful.

Vegetable Soup II

Gently boil vegetables of your choice for two minutes. Take the vegetables out, save the broth, and blend vegetables in a blender. Return pureed vegetables to the broth and reheat.

Simple Bean Soup

> *2 cans beans of your choice*
> *Celery*
> *Cooking wine (optional)*
> *Soy sauce*
> *Salt*
> *Orange peel*
> *Butter*
> *Half-and-half cream*
> *Cinnamon*

In a large saucepan, heat the beans (including the liquid), diced celery, and additional water as needed. Bring to a boil. Add a splash of wine and soy sauce, salt to taste, and a small amount of orange peel diced very fine. Boil gently for about ten to fifteen minutes. Add a tablespoon or two of butter and half-and-half. Simmer for a few more minutes, add a few dashes of cinnamon and serve.

Bone Soup

> 1½ lbs. of bones
> 5 small- to medium-sized potatoes, cut into cubes
> 8–12 cherry or small plum tomatoes, cut into pieces
> ½–1 medium-sized fennel bulb, chopped (fennel fans add more!)
> 5–6 cups of water
> Approximately ½ cup cooking wine
> Oil to sauté vegetables (2–3 tablespoons)
> A pinch or two of cinnamon
> Salt (to taste)
> (You can be creative and use other vegetables such as carrots, celery, mushrooms, string beans, and onions.)

Rinse the bones and set aside. In a 4–5 quart stockpot, sauté the potatoes, tomatoes, and fennel (and any other vegetables you add to the soup) in oil. (Sautéing vegetables first keeps them from turning mushy in the soup.) Add bones, water, wine, and spices. Bring to a boil slowly. Turn down heat and let soup simmer for several hours, stirring occasionally. Remove bones (you can scoop out any marrow remaining in the hollow of bones and add to soup) and serve soup hot. (This recipe can also be made in a crockpot.)

*Supermarkets frequently sell packages of bones for soup, but the best bet is to go to your local butcher shop and ask for bones—they sometimes even give them away. Thigh bones are preferable because they contain the most marrow. A whole thigh bone (beef) yields about six pounds of bone. You can request only a few pounds or take the rest home and freeze it for future use. Have the butcher cut the bone into 3-inch–4-inch sections so it easily fits into the pot and also exposes more of the marrow.

Walnuts and Black Sesame Seeds

> ½ pound walnuts
> ½ pound black sesame seeds
> 3–4 ounces honey

Grind ingredients together in a blender. Cook in a double boiler or steam for one hour. After cooking, refrigerate. Eat two table-spoons in the morning and two in the evening. This high-energy treat benefits the kidney, spleen, liver, and lung; it is also espe-cially good for the skin and hair.

Fresh Royal Jelly and Bee Pollen

These bee products are high in energy and safe to take every day. Fresh royal jelly is the food given to a queen bee by her workers. It enables her to live for up to five years (as opposed to about three months for the drones) and to produce twice her weight in eggs every day. It is better to take the fresh jelly, not the capsules. It's not very tasty, so you can mix ½–1 teaspoon of the jelly with honey and a little warm water. Drink this once a day.

Bee pollen can also be taken once a day, and again, because of the taste you will probably want to mix it with honey and warm water. Take 1–2 teaspoons (separately from the fresh royal jelly—don't mix the two together).

Ginseng

Ginseng increases Qi and is very good for treating hot flashes nat-urally. It should, however, be treated as a medicine and not as something that is good for anyone at anytime. Don't take it if you are under fifty, and healthy—ginseng adds too much Qi from an external source, and makes your own Qi, or vital energy, lazy. If you take ginseng for menopausal symptoms, be sure it is Chinese or Korean ginseng of good quality. You can take it in capsule form, but it is best to use the whole root.

Boil about a handful of the roots in a quart of water, and then let them simmer for about two hours. You can use a double-boiler, crockpot, or a special Chinese ginseng cooker which is similar to a double boiler. Take one or two glasses a day on an empty stomach. You can cook the same roots four times, and eat the roots themselves after the last cooking.

If you experience any uncomfortable side effects from ginseng, such as insomnia or palpitations, you should stop taking it. These symptoms indicate that ginseng is not good for you, and you should consult a doctor knowledgeable in herbal therapy.

Chicken and Ginseng

> *Small baby or spring chicken*
> *2 slices fresh ginger*
> *Pinch of cinnamon*
> *1.5 ounces ginseng*
> *1 tablespoon, cooking wine (optional)*
> *Salt and pepper to taste*

Start with a small baby or spring chicken. Add two slices of fresh ginger and a little bit of cinnamon. Add ginseng. If desired, add one tablespoon of cooking wine. Put all ingredients together in one pot. Cover with water to a depth of about two inches above the chicken. Bring to a boil; then let simmer for about an hour. Another way to cook this dish is to put all the ingredients in a crockpot, adding boiling water to two inches above the chicken. Simmer all day. When you're ready to eat, salt to taste. Eat this dish at least twice a week.

This dish can also be prepared with beef, lamb, or pork bone. If you're a vegetarian, cook the ginseng as above without meat and drink one cup of the liquid as a tea twice a day for at least a week.

Herbal Healing Pad

> *2–3 ounces each of the following:*
> *Dried ginger*
> *Clove*
> *Cinnamon*
> *Fennel*
> *Tangerine peel*

Put all the ingredients in a small cloth bag or pillow, and steam or microwave until warm. If you use a microwave, make sure the cloth is 100 percent cotton. Place this bag on the lower abdomen, about the width of four fingers below your belly button (This is point *Guanyuan*) or the small of the back (point *Mingmen*). Heating these areas will help increase Qi and will also help relieve symptoms such as cramps, PMS, and stomachache. You can reuse the same bag several times, until there is no longer an aroma from the warmed ingredients.

HEALING HERBS FOR MENOPAUSE

Classical Chinese herbs and herbal formulas work from the inside. Similar to acupuncture, herbs are good for problems relating to the function of an organ (although their effect is more indirect); they are also very good for physical problems. The Qi of herbs is absorbed by the body, and it works to strengthen and balance any organ that is weak or out of order. Chinese herbs are very powerful medicine and should be prescribed by a knowledgeable TCM practitioner or herbalist.

The purpose of this section is not self-diagnosis or self-treatment. It's impossible to read a book and try to figure out on your own what herbs you need. In the case of traditional Chinese medicine, you may even make your condition worse. We've seen how TCM approaches treatment on the basis of the individual. You can't assume that herb A is good for condition B, because the same symptoms can arise from different causes. Herbal prescriptions should change as you do, and for this too the guidance of a good practitioner is necessary.

The Qi of each herb used in TCM goes to a particular meridian where it supports the function of the corresponding organ. This knowledge has been used for many centuries to heal millions and millions of people. I've created a reference guide in Chapter 15 so that you can learn more about TCM herbs for treating the symptoms of menopause. This way you can educate yourself and have more knowledge to work effectively with your herbalist or TCM doctor. This practitioner must know not only which herbs to use, but how much, and in what combination with other herbs to maximize their effect. Herbs work best as a team, and putting that team together requires knowledge, skill, sensitivity, and even artistry. A wrong combination of herbs can do more harm than good. Your herbalist must also know how to cook a particular prescription, as the cooking method changes the effect of the herbs. He or she must be able to recognize any side effects of herbal therapy, which can be quite subtle (another good reason to avoid self-prescribing herbs).

Here are a number of herbs that have been used, in some cases, for thousands of years by TCM practitioners to help women go through menopause naturally. As with the foods and recipes above, I have selected those that are best for Western women. The herbs are listed with their alternate English names, as well as their Latin names and Pinyin designations. (Pinyin is the system used to transform Chinese characters into words that can be pronounced.) Each of these entries also identifies the essence of the herb, the meridian or meridians it affects, as well as how the herb helps the body and which conditions it can improve. Dosages listed here are for average usage. When a condition changes, the TCM practitioner adjusts the dosage accordingly. In my practice, I use a number of these herbs frequently as key ingredients in special herbal formulations that I've developed to help Western women with menopausal symptoms.

Remember we discussed earlier how TCM uses herbs. Most are used in the context of a team of herbs with each one assigned a specific role; some can be used singly or in small combinations. The Chinese pride themselves on being inventive and efficient.

They like to kill two birds with one stone. So they have an entire portion of Chinese healing arts devoted to combining foods and herbs together for the purpose of healing. This is known as *"shi liao,"* which means using food for healing purposes, or *"yao shan,"* which means using herbs as food to heal. Some herbs can be cooked together with other foods such as chicken, fish, pork, or lamb to enhance their effects. There are actually a number of well-known restaurants in China and Hong Kong that serve meals of this kind. Here, you can describe your condition to the waiters and they will recommend the proper healing foods to order.

Astragalus Root

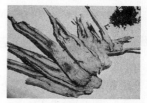

ALTERNATE ENGLISH NAME: None
LATIN NAME: *Radix Astragali seu Hedysari*
PINYIN: *Huang qi, Jin qi*
FLAVOR: Sweet
ESSENCE: Warm
MERIDIANS: Enters the spleen and lung meridians
EFFECTS
- Strengthens the immune system
- Tones and boosts Qi
- Diuretic
- Disperses swelling
- Detoxifies

INDICATIONS:
- Deficiency of Qi or vital energy, manifesting as symptoms of increased susceptibility to colds and flu, numbness in the extremities, spontaneous sweating, bleeding from uterus, blood in stool
- Spleen function problems (which can involve symptoms such as poor appetite, loose stool, lethargy)
- Prolapse of organs
- Skin problems/infections such as sores, carbuncles, boils

- Diabetes

DOSAGE: 10–15 grams, 30–60 grams for a large dosage, decocted in water for an oral dose

Astragalus Tonic

Many Chinese herb stores now have a tonic with astragalus. This tonic is particularly good for those with chronic fatigue or after surgery, chemotherapy, and radiation.

Angelica Root

ALTERNATE ENGLISH NAME: *Dong quai,* tangkuei root, Chinese Angelica root

LATIN NAME: *Radix Angelicae sinensis*

PINYIN: *Dang gui*

FLAVOR: Sweet and pungent

ESSENCE: Warm

MERIDIANS: Enters the liver, heart, and spleen meridians

EFFECTS

- Tones the blood (builds T-cells), increases blood circulation
- Relieves pain
- Moistens the bowels
- Regulates menstruation

INDICATIONS:

- A condition of blood deficiency (such as that after surgery, cancer treatment; often manifesting with symptoms of pale lips and tongue, sallow complexion, dizziness, palpitations)
- Irregular menstruation (absence of periods, painful periods), uterine bleeding
- Various pains due to stagnation of blood, rheumatic joint pain, impact injuries
- Constipation
- Skin infections, sores, carbuncles, boils

DOSAGE: 5-15 grams, decocted in water for an oral dose.

NOTES: Stir-frying Angelica root with wine increases its properties of promoting menstrual flow and increasing blood circulation.

This root is often used together with astragalus to replenish the blood.

Chinese Angelica root should not be used in cases of excessive dampness manifesting in abdominal distention and loose stool.

Bupleurum Root

ALTERNATIVE ENGLISH NAME: Honey root
LATIN NAME: *Radix bupleuri*
PINYIN: *Chai hu*
FLAVOR: Bitter and pungent
ESSENCE: Cold
MERIDIANS: Liver and gallbladder
EFFECTS
- Helps smooth liver function
- Promotes the flow of Qi
- Reduces fever and conditions of internal heat

INDICATIONS
- Often used for chills and fever that come and go
- Bitter taste in the mouth
- Chest tightness
- Menstrual cycle irregularities
- Liver Qi stagnation
- Conditions of collapse—either of Qi or organs like the uterus

DOSAGE: 3–10 grams

Chinese Yam Rhizome

ALTERNATE ENGLISH NAME: Dioscorea rhizome
LATIN NAME: *Rhizoma Dioscoreae*
PINYIN: *Shan yao, Huai shan yao*
FLAVOR: Sweet
ESSENCE: Neutral
MERIDIANS: Enters the spleen, lung, and kidney meridians
EFFECTS
- Strengthens the kidney

- Improves the function of the spleen and stomach
- Promotes production of body fluids to nourish the lung

INDICATIONS

- Deficiency of the kidney (which can manifest in symptoms such as frequent urination, vaginal discharge)
- Digestive problems such as poor appetite, loose stool, or diarrhea
- Cough, shortness of breath
- Diabetes, loss of body fluids, thirst

DOSAGE: 10–30 grams, large dosage 60–250 grams, decocted in water for an oral dose; or ground into powder for an oral administration: 6–10 grams each time

PRECAUTIONS: Chinese yam should not be used in cases of abdominal distention due to excessive dampness or stagnant food.

Cinnamon Bark

ALTERNATE ENGLISH NAME: None

LATIN NAME: *Cortex Cinnamomi*

PINYIN: *Rou gui*

FLAVOR: Pungent and sweet

ESSENCE: Hot

MERIDIANS: Enters the kidney, spleen, liver, and heart meridians

EFFECTS

- Helps kidney function
- Gets rid of cold conditions in the body
- Relieves pain
- Warms up and promotes flow of energy through the meridians

INDICATIONS

- Cold conditions such as cold limbs, feelings of aversion to cold
- Frequent urination
- Various pains (such as knee pain, lumbago)
- Gastric and abdominal pain, poor appetite, loose stool

- Menstrual problems such as painful periods, absence of periods, abnormal clotting
- Skin sores, abscesses, carbuncles, boils

DOSAGE: 2–5 grams, decocted later than other drugs when prepared for a decoction; 1–2 grams ground into a powder for an infusion taken orally

Cistanche Herb

ALTERNATE ENGLISH NAME: None
LATIN NAME: *Herba Cistanchis*
PINYIN: *Rou cong rong*
FLAVOR: Sweet and salty
ESSENCE: Warm
MERIDIANS: Kidney and large intestine
EFFECTS

- Strengthens kidney Qi
- Invigorates or tonifies blood and increases blood volume
- Moistens the large intestine and helps relieve constipation

INDICATIONS

- Kidney Qi deficiency
- Lower back pain
- Fatigue
- Infertility in women
- Constipation
- Hot flashes

Codonopsis Root

ALTERNATIVE ENGLISH NAME: None
Latin NAME: *Radix Codonopsis pilosulae*
PINYIN: *Dang shen*
FLAVOR: Sweet
ESSENCE: Neutral
MERIDIANS: Enters the spleen and lung meridians
EFFECTS

- Tones the spleen and lung
- Promotes the production of blood and body fluids

- Increases Qi

INDICATIONS

- For conditions of spleen Qi deficiencies including prolapse of stomach, uterus, kidney, and rectum
- For menstrual irregularities and blood deficiencies
- Dizziness, shortness of breath

This herb has also been used recently in China for insomnia and other sleeping disorders, anemia, excessive uterine bleeding, and bruising.

DOSAGE: 9–30 grams

Coix Seed

ALTERNATE ENGLISH NAME: Job's tears seed

LATIN NAME: *Semen Coicis*

PINYIN: *Yi ren mi, Yi mi ren*

FLAVOR: Bland and sweet

ESSENCE: Cold

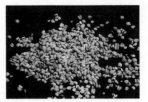

MERIDIANS: Enters the spleen, lung, and kidney meridians

EFFECTS

- Strengthens the spleen
- Strengthens the lung
- Eliminates dampness from the body
- Relieves the body of excess internal heat

INDICATIONS

- Obstruction of meridians, particularly by dampness
- Arthritic pain (due to dampness), muscular spasm in the limbs
- Edema
- Diarrhea
- Weakness of the lungs
- Vaginal discharge

DOSAGE: 10–30 grams, decocted in water for an oral dose

Coix Seed Breakfast Dish

This herb is particularly good for preventing cancer. It can help strengthen your digestive system and help rid the body of edema, or excess water. It is also useful for helping reduce arthritis pain. You can cook this as a breakfast dish.

> 1 cup of Coix seed
> 1 cup of Lotus seed
> 1 cup of Chinese red dates

You can also add raw peanuts to this dish. Put ingredients in a pot and add two quarts of water. Bring to a boil and then simmer for about forty minutes until the mixture cooks down. You can sweeten to taste with honey or brown sugar. This dish makes enough for about five days. You can cook it ahead of time and re-heat each morning. You can add more water, or soy or regular milk, if you prefer a thinner consistency.

PRECAUTIONS: Use with care in pregnancy.

Corn Silk

ALTERNATE ENGLISH NAME: Zea, Maydis, Stigmata
LATIN NAME: *Stigma maydis*
PINYIN: *Yu mi xu*
FLAVOR: Sweet
ESSENCE: Neutral
MERIDIANS: Enters the liver, gallbladder, stomach, and urinary bladder meridians
EFFECTS

- Relieves water, dampness, and heat in the body
- Helps the gallbladder to pass stones (classically, in traditional Chinese medicine, corn silk has been prescribed for kidney stones and diabetes in addition to gallstones)
- Helps digestive system function well, particularly good for stomach and liver problems

INDICATIONS
- Edema and swelling in the body
- Excess internal heat
- Gallstones
- Digestive disturbances such as diarrhea, belching, nausea

DOSAGE: 30–150 grams, decocted in water for an oral dose

Corn Silk Tea

Save the silk from ears of corn and dry it. Take a handful of corn silk (about 20 grams) and boil in 3 cups water until the liquid has been reduced by half. Drink tea while it is hot. Drink twice a day.

Curculiginis

ALTERNATE ENGLISH NAME: None
LATIN NAME: *Rhizoma Curculiginis*
PINYIN: *Xian mao*
FLAVOR: Pungent
ESSENCE: Warm
MERIDIANS: Kidney, liver, and spleen

EFFECTS
- Strengthens kidney Qi
- Strengthens spleen Qi
- Strengthens tendons and bones
- Expels internal cold and dampness

INDICATIONS
- Kidney and spleen Qi deficiencies
- Urinary frequency
- Incontinence
- Hormone imbalances
- Arthritis pain due to dampness
- Fatigue
- Poor appetite
- Diarrhea
- Abdominal pain

- Hot flashes and night sweats

DOSAGE: 9–12 grams

Dolichos Seed

ALTERNATE ENGLISH NAME:
Lablab seed

LATIN NAME: *Semen Dolichoris seu Lablab*

PINYIN: *Bian dou*

FLAVOR: Sweet

ESSENCE: Slightly warm

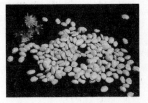

MERIDIANS: Enters the spleen and stomach meridians

EFFECTS

- Strengthens Qi
- Balances digestive organs
- Relieves dampness in the body

INDICATIONS

- Vomiting, diarrhea related to dampness climatic conditions
- Thirst, increased fluid intake, frequent urination, diabetes
- Poor appetite
- Vaginal discharge (both red and white)

DOSAGE: 5–12 grams, decocted in water for a daily dose

Epimedium

ALTERNATE ENGLISH NAME: Epimedium herb

LATIN NAME: *Herba Epimedii*

PINYIN: *Yin yang huo*

FLAVOR: Sweet and pungent

ESSENCE: Warm

MERIDIANS: Enters the liver and kidney meridians

EFFECTS

- Strengthens kidney Qi
- Strengthens tendons and bones
- Relieves wind and dampness

INDICATIONS
- Weak kidney function
- Lower back pain and weakness of the knees
- High blood pressure
- Hot flashes and night sweats
- Infertility in women
- Frequent urination
- Impotence

DOSAGE: 9–15 grams

Eucommia Bark

ALTERNATE ENGLISH NAME: None
LATIN NAME: *Cortex Eucommiae*
PINYIN: *Du zhong*
FLAVOR: Warm and sweet
MERIDIANS: Liver and kidney
EFFECTS
- Nourishes the liver and kidney
- Strengthens bones and muscles. Prevents miscarriage
- Relieves excessive bleeding from the vagina or uterus

INDICATIONS
- High blood pressure
- Tinnitus or ringing in the ears
- Kidney Qi deficiency
- Urinary frequency

DOSAGE: 10–15 grams

Germinated Barley

ALTERNATE ENGLISH NAME: Dried barley sprout, malt
LATIN NAME: *Fructus Hordei germinates*
PINYIN: *Mai ya*
FLAVOR: Sweet and mild
ESSENCE: Neutral
MERIDIANS: Enters the stomach, spleen, and liver meridians
EFFECTS
- Tones the digestive system

- Stops milk production in lactating women
- Helps liver function smoothly

INDICATIONS
- Digestive system problems (for example, lactose and/or wheat intolerance, poor appetite, indigestion, food retention)
- Breast pain (a distending pain), to stop milk secretion

DOSAGE: 30–130 grams, decocted in water for an oral dose

The following recipe is very good for anyone who wants to keep their stomach function strong. It is also good for individuals who already have a digestive system problem, PMS, breast tenderness, or wheat or milk allergies. In my opinion, germinated barley offers much more benefit than wheatgrass. Use this herb as a tea or as a breakfast cereal.

Germinated Barley Recipes

Germinated barley may be difficult to find, but here's a simple way you can make your own. Buy a bag of organic barley. Soak in water overnight. Then strain the water and spread the barley evenly about one-inch thick in an aluminum pan. Cover with a wet towel and keep in a warm place. Spray with water twice a day. Based on your room temperature, it should take about two days to germinate or sprout. When the sprouts reach about one inch in length, the barley is ready to be dried for use. One way to dry the sprouts is to put them in a slow oven around 140 degrees. Do not use high heat, which will destroy the healing benefits of the barley. After drying, store in an airtight container.

Germinated Barley Tea

2 handfuls (around 6 grams) germinated barley
1–2 pieces fresh ginger
2 slices tangerine peels

Take germinated barley, add fresh ginger, and tangerine peels, if available. Put in a pot and cover with one quart of water. Bring to a boil; then simmer for about twenty minutes. Strain this mixture and drink the water as a tea.

Germinated Barley Cereal

Another way to use germinated barley is to soak it overnight, then put it in a blender. Follow the above recipe until the boiling stage. Now you have an oatmeal-like mixture that you can eat for breakfast. You can add sesame seeds, peanuts, walnuts, or any other kind of nuts, to enhance the flavor and healing benefits. Sweeten with honey and add cinnamon to taste.

PRECAUTIONS: Germinated barley should not be used by women who are breast-feeding.

Ginkgo Leaf
ALTERNATE ENGLISH NAME: None
LATIN NAME: *Folium Ginko*
PINYIN: *Bae guo ye*
FLAVOR: Sweet and slightly bitter
ESSENCE: Neutral
MERIDIANS: Enters the lung and stomach meridians
EFFECTS
- Relieves pain
- Nourishes lung, relieves cough
- Promotes general circulation
- Helps heart disease
INDICATIONS
- High cholesterol, high blood pressure, palpitations
- Coughs (any kind of cough)
DOSAGE: 3–6 grams, decocted in water; 500–1000 milligrams, powdered form in capsule for a daily dose

Ginseng (American)
ALTERNATE ENGLISH NAME: Man's health, tartar root, five fingers

LATIN NAME: *Radix Panacis Quinquefolii*
PINYIN: *Xi yang shen*
FLAVOR: Sweet and slightly bitter
ESSENCE: Neutral
MERIDIANS: Enters the heart, lung, and kidney meridians
EFFECTS
- Tones Qi and blood
- Relieves heat in body
- Promotes production of body fluids
INDICATIONS
- Lung problems, especially heat in lung, cough (all kinds)
- Loss of fluids and blood (e.g., during chemotherapy, radiation, after surgery)
- Constipation
DOSAGE: 500–1000 milligrams powder in capsule form for daily use

Ginseng (Chinese)

ALTERNATE ENGLISH NAME: Ginseng root, white ginseng
LATIN NAME: *Radix Ginseng*
PINYIN: *Ren shen*
FLAVOR: Sweet and slightly bitter
ESSENCE: Neutral
MERIDIANS: Enters the spleen, lung, and heart meridians
EFFECTS
- Increases Qi, in this case, particularly "original" Qi, which forms the basis of kidney Qi
- Tones the spleen and lung
- Promotes production of blood and body fluids
- Calms the spirit
- Improves mental power
INDICATIONS
- Depleted Qi or vital energy which can produce symptoms such as shortness of breath, listlessness, weak pulse; especially after a severe or prolonged illness

- A large loss of blood (such as that caused by childbirth, uterine bleeding, or traumatic injuries)
- Digestive disturbances such as loss of appetite, diarrhea
- Lung problems such as cough, shortness of breath
- Loss of body fluids (due to symptoms like spontaneous sweating, frequent urination, such as occurs in diabetes)
- Heart problems (with symptoms like palpitations)
- Insomnia, dream-disturbed sleep, irritability

DOSAGE: 5–10 grams, decocted alone with low heat and its decoction mixed with that of other herbs for an oral dose; 1–2 grams of ginseng root ground into powder and taken in capsule form 2–3 times per day; 15–30 grams for a large dosage.

Ginseng is the one herb that can increase Qi quickly. It can be used individually or in combination with foods or other herbs.

PRECAUTIONS: Ginseng should not be used in conjunction with black hellebore, trogopterus dung, and honey locust; tea and radish should be avoided during the time ginseng is used to avoid reducing its efficacy. TCM does *not* recommend taking ginseng for the common cold.

Ginseng (Siberian)

ALTERNATE ENGLISH NAME: Siberian ginseng, Eleuthero ginseng
LATIN NAME: *Radix Acanthopanacis Senticosi*
PINYIN NAME: *Ci wu jia*
FLAVOR: Bitter and pungent
ESSENCE: Warm
MERIDIANS: Enters the liver and kidney meridians
EFFECTS

- Increases Qi or vital energy
- Nourishes the heart and helps tranquilize the mind
- Expels wind and dampness
- Strengthens tendons and bones

INDICATIONS
- Increases spleen Qi, helps loose stool, fatigue, poor appetite
- Nourishes the heart Qi, helps insomnia, and palpitations
- For chronic rheumatism with weakness of extremities, infantile paralysis

DOSAGE: 6–15 grams. Tablet form: 2–4 tablets

Recently, Siberian ginseng has been used for leukocytopenia and coronary heart disease, chronic bronchitis, thromboangiitis obliterans. Often used as complementary treatment with cancer drugs or x-ray therapy for tumors.

*American ginseng is also good for menopausal symptoms

Glehnia Root
ALTERNATE ENGLISH NAME: None
LATIN NAME: *Radix Glehniae*
PINYIN: *Sha shen*
FLAVOR: Sweet
ESSENCE: Slightly cold
MERIDIANS: Enters the lung and stomach meridians
EFFECTS
- Clears heat from the lung
- Nourishes yin Qi
- Strengthens stomach function
- Promotes the production of body fluids
INDICATIONS
- Conditions such as a dry cough caused by heat in the lung
- Lack of body fluids due to a fever

Hawthorn Berry
ALTERNATE ENGLISH NAME:
Crataegus fruit, redhaw fruit
LATIN NAME: *Fructus Crataegi*
PINYIN: *Shan zha*
FLAVOR: Sour and sweet
ESSENCE: Slightly warm

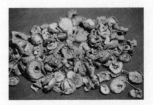

MERIDIANS: Enters the spleen, stomach, and liver meridians
EFFECTS
- Improves digestion
- Disperses and removes stagnant food
- Increases blood circulation, removes blood stagnation
- Expels tapeworm

INDICATIONS
- Indigestion and retention of food (due to improper diet of too much greasy food and/or meat), symptoms of loss of appetite, abdominal distention, abdominal pain, diarrhea
- Masses, tumors (breast masses and/or tumors)
- Heart disease (angina pectoris, hypertension)
- Postpartum difficulties (pain, abnormal flow of lochia)

DOSAGE: 10–15 grams, 30–60 grams for a large dosage, decocted in water for an oral dose

Licorice Root

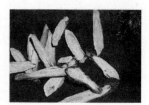

ALTERNATE ENGLISH NAME: None
LATIN NAME: *Radix Glycyrrhizae*
PINYIN: *Gan cao*
FLAVOR: Sweet
ESSENCE: Neutral
MERIDIANS: Enters the heart, lung, spleen, and stomach meridians
EFFECTS
- Increases Qi or overall vital energy
- Tones the function of the spleen
- Relieves body of internal heat
- Detoxifies
- Relieves pain and spasm
- Harmonizes the properties of other herbs

INDICATIONS
- Spleen function problems involving poor appetite, diarrhea
- Cough, shortness of breath
- Skin infections such as sores, carbuncles, and boils
- Sore throat

- Food poisoning
- Stomachache, abdominal pain, muscular spasm and pain, spasm and pain in the extremities

DOSAGE: 2–10 grams, as the principal herb

There is a famous herbal formula recipe that has been in use since the Sung Dynasty (960-1127 A.D.), which the Chinese call *Si Jun Zi Tang*. It combines licorice with ginseng, poria, and white atractylodes rhizome. Though it only uses four herbs, each one has a specific and unique healing role. This formula has been used for almost a thousand years to help increase the body's Qi and improve the function of the stomach and spleen.

This herbal formula is especially good for anyone with a poor digestive system, loose stool, lack of appetite, and fatigue. It can also help those recovering from surgery, chemotherapy, and radiation treatment. This classical formula can be bought at many Chinese herb stores. It forms the basis of a number of other classical Chinese herbal formulas that have helped millions over many centuries. Follow the directions on the box. (If you cannot find this formula locally, it can be ordered from our Foundation; see the contact information in the Appendix. I have adapted a series of formulas for my Western patients. They are called BCPP— Breast Cancer Prevention Project—Herbal Master.)

PRECAUTIONS: Licorice root is not to be used with kansui root, knoxia root, and genkwa flower; if licorice root is taken in large doses over a long period of time, it can possibly cause edema.

Lily Bulb

ALTERNATE ENGLISH NAME: None
LATIN NAME: *Bulbus Lilii*
PINYIN: *Bai he*
FLAVOR: Sweet and slightly bitter
ESSENCE: Slightly cold
MERIDIANS: Enters the lung and heart meridians

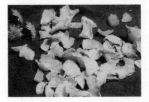

EFFECTS

- Nourishes the lung, moistens the lung, arrests cough
- Balances heart function, clears "fire" in the heart to quiet the spirit
- Gets rid of excess water in the body

INDICATIONS

- Cough due to dryness of the lung, tubercular cough with sputum in blood
- Fever conditions, especially lingering fever
- Insomnia, clouded thinking
- Heart palpitations, especially stimulated by strong emotions
- Edema

DOSAGE: 10–30 grams, decocted in water for an oral dose

Motherwort

ALTERNATE ENGLISH NAME: Chinese motherwort, leonurus
LATIN NAME: *Herba Leonuri*
PINYIN: *Yi mu cao*
FLAVOR: Pungent and bitter
ESSENCE: Slightly cold
MERIDIANS: Enters the heart, liver, and urinary bladder meridians

EFFECTS

- Diuretic
- Increases blood circulation, removes blood stagnation
- Clears internal heat from body
- Detoxifies
- Improves cardiovascular health

INDICATIONS

- Edema, difficulty in urinating
- Irregular or stagnant menstruation, absence of menstruation
- Postpartum abdominal pain
- Distending pain in lower abdomen
- Sports injuries, traumatic injuries with pain and swelling
- Skin sores, infections
- Heart disease such as angina pectoris

DOSAGE: 10–15 grams decocted in water for an oral dose; for inducing diuresis to treat edema, the large dosage can be 30–60 grams

NOTES: Used externally on skin sores, infections

PRECAUTIONS: It should not be used in cases of deficiency of blood without blood stasis.

Notoginseng Root

ALTERNATE ENGLISH NAME: Notoginseng, Sanchi root

LATIN NAME: *Radix Notoginseng*

PINYIN: *San qi*

FLAVOR: Sweet and slightly bitter

ESSENCE: Warm

MERIDIANS: Enters the liver and stomach meridians

EFFECTS

- Increases blood flow (circulation) and also stops bleeding
- Helps the function of the heart and liver
- Increases Qi without the side effects associated with Chinese or American (or other types of) ginseng
- Relieves insomnia, palpitations
- Relieves pain
- Reduces swelling, inflammation, masses, tumors

INDICATIONS

- Various types of internal bleeding (such as uterine bleeding, coughing up of blood, blood in stool) and external bleeding (for example, due to traumatic injuries)
- Heart disease (such as angina pectoris)
- Sports injuries
- Breast masses, tumors, other types of masses and tumors

DOSAGE: 1–3 grams, ground into powder for swallowing (2000–3000 milligrams daily, powder in capsules); "proper amount" for external use

NOTES: If you have blood stagnation, which can appear as clotting during the menstrual cycle, have blue marks on the side of your tongue, bruise easily, suffer from cardiovascular disease or varicose veins, or you've had a sports injury, notoginseng is one of the best herbs you can take.

The following is an example of combining foods and herbs for a healing dish:

Chicken with Notoginseng

> 1 ounce notoginseng
> 2 teaspoons cooking wine
> 4 pieces of scallion
> Small baby or spring chicken
> Salt

Combine notoginseng with cooking wine. Put 4 pieces of scallion with small baby or spring chicken in a pot. Cover with water to a depth of 2 inches above the chicken. Bring ingredients to a boil. Simmer for an hour. Salt to taste before eating.

Notoginseng Tea

Today, you can find notoginseng tea in some Chinese herb stores. It is an excellent blood tonic. Drink it daily to help prevent heart disease. (If you cannot find it locally, you can order it through our Foundation. See the contact information in the back of this book.)

Oldenlandia

ALTERNATE ENGLISH NAME: None

LATIN NAME: *Herba Oldenlandia diffusa*

PINYIN: *Bai hua she she cao*

FLAVOR: Bitter and sweet

ESSENCE: Cold

MERIDIANS: Enters the stomach, large intestine, and small intestine meridians

EFFECTS

- Relieves/reduces heat in the body
- Relieves internal conditions of dampness
- Shrinks masses and tumors

- Detoxifies internal poisons (Oldenlandia has been used classically in TCM both internally and externally to treat poisons, e.g., snakebite)

INDICATIONS

- Cancer
- Various forms of poisoning or conditions where toxins have built up in the body
- Masses, tumors

DOSAGE: 15-60 grams, decocted in water for an oral dose

Oldenlandia Tea

Many Chinese herb stores carry Oldenlandia in powdered form, from which you can make a tea. Drink a cup or two every other day to help detoxify your system. (If you cannot find this herb locally, you can order the tea from our Foundation. See the contact information in the back of this book.)

Polygonum Root

ALTERNATE ENGLISH NAME: Polygonum root
LATIN NAME: *Radix Polygonia multiflori*
PINYIN NAME: *He shou wu*
FLAVOR: Bittersweet and pungent
ESSENCE: Warm
MERIDIAN: Liver and kidney meridians

EFFECTS

- Strengthens liver function and kidney Qi
- Helps blood deficiency
- Relaxes the bowels
- Detoxifies the whole body

INDICATIONS

- Graying of the hair or hair loss
- Palpitations, dizziness, tinnitus
- Blurred vision
- Insomnia
- Lower back pain, weakness or numbness in the knees
- Constipation

DOSAGE: 15–30 grams

This herb has recently been used for hypercholesterinemia and atherosclerosis.

Poria

ALTERNATE ENGLISH NAME: Hoelen, tuckahoe
LATIN NAME: *Poria (Hoelen)*
PINYIN: *Fu ling*
FLAVOR: Sweet, tasteless in flavor
ESSENCE: Neutral
MERIDIANS: Enters heart, spleen, and kidney meridians
EFFECTS
- Tones the spleen
- Diuretic (rids body of excess water, fluids; excretes dampness)
- Tranquilizes the spirit

INDICATIONS
- Urinary tract problems such as painful or difficult urination, infections
- Edema (retention of fluids in the body)
- Excess phlegm, cough
- Digestive disturbances such as loss of appetite, loose stool
- Heart problems (which can result in symptoms like palpitations)
- Insomnia, fatigue, dizziness

DOSAGE: 10–15 grams, decocted in water for an oral dose

NOTES: This root is sticky and greasy in nature and can hinder digestion, so it should not be used if digestion is poor.

Prunella

ALTERNATE ENGLISH NAME: Self-heal, heal-all
LATIN NAME: *Spica Prunellae*
PINYIN: *Xia ku cao*
FLAVOR: Bitter, acrid
ESSENCE: Cold
MERIDIANS: Enters the liver and gallbladder meridians

EFFECTS
- Helps the liver to function smoothly
- Breaks up lumps and masses

INDICATIONS
- Lumps, masses, tumors in the body
- Goiter (swelling of the thyroid gland)
- Mammary abscess
- Excess tearing of the eyes and aversion to light, eyeball pain (especially at night)
- Sinew and bone pain
- Pulmonary tuberculosis
- Acute icteric (jaundice) infectious hepatitis
- Uterine bleeding

DOSAGE: 3–10 grams, decocted in water for an oral dose

Prunella Tea

Prunella tea is good for reducing tumors and helping skin problems. You can buy this at most Chinese herb stores. Put 2 ounces of the herb in 2 quarts of water. Bring to a boil. Let simmer for about thirty minutes. You can drink this tea once or twice a day as part of your daily self-healing regimen.

Prunella and Oldenlandia Tea

These two herbs in combination have been used effectively by many TCM doctors to treat cancer and tumors. If you have cancer, you can combine one ounce of prunella with one ounce of oldenlandia to make a tea that can be very useful during chemotherapy and radiation.

Psoralea Fruit

ALTERNATE ENGLISH NAME: None
LATIN NAME: *Fructus Psoraleae*
PINYIN: *Bu gu zhi*
FLAVOR: Pungent and bitter
ESSENCE: Warm
MERIDIANS: Enters the spleen and kidney meridians

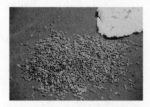

EFFECTS
- Helps kidney function

INDICATIONS
- Lumbago
- Frequent urination
- Pain in the loins and knees (of a cold type)
- Cough, shortness of breath

DOSAGE: 5–10 grams, decocted in water for an oral dose, or used in pills or powder form

Red Sage Root

ALTERNATE ENGLISH NAME: Red-rooted sage, salvia root
LATIN NAME: *Radix Salviae miltiorrhizae*
PINYIN: *Dan shen*
FLAVOR: Bitter
ESSENCE: Slightly cold
MERIDIANS: Enters the heart, pericardium, and liver meridians

EFFECTS
- Increases blood circulation, nourishes (builds up) the blood (increases blood cells), relieves heat in the blood
- Calms the spirit

INDICATIONS
- Menstrual problems such as PMS, painful periods, irregular periods; obstetrical problems
- Skin sores, carbuncles, boils
- Stomach and abdominal pain
- Masses in the abdomen
- Insomnia, irritability, palpitations

DOSAGE: 5–15 grams, decocted in water for an oral dose
PRECAUTIONS: Antagonistic to black hellebore rhizome

Rehmannia Root (Cooked)

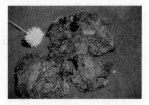

ALTERNATE ENGLISH NAME: None
LATIN NAME: *Radix Rehmanniae Praeparata*
PINYIN NAME: *Shu di*

FLAVOR: Sweet and slightly bitter
ESSENCE: Slightly warm
MERIDIANS: Enters the heart, liver, and kidney meridians
EFFECTS
- Strengthens liver and kidney functions
- Nourishes body fluids and moisturizes conditions of dryness
- Increases kidney Qi and enriches blood
INDICATIONS
- Lower back pain with aching knees
- Osteoarthritis
- Hot flashes and night sweats
- Fatigue, dizziness, palpitations
DOSAGE: 10–30 grams

NOTES: This herb has recently been used for hypertension and hypercholesterinemia.

Safflower

ALTERNATE ENGLISH NAME:
Carthamus flower
LATIN NAME: *Flos Carthami*
PINYIN: *Hong hua*
FLAVOR: Pungent
ESSENCE: Warm

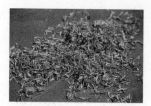

MERIDIANS: Enters the heart and liver meridians
EFFECTS
- Increases blood circulation
- Eliminates blood stagnation
- Normalizes menstruation
- Breaks up masses
- Helps reduce body pains caused by stagnation of blood
INDICATIONS
- Menstrual difficulties, including PMS, irregular periods, painful periods, absence of periods, "scanty" periods
- Postpartum pain, pain in lower abdomen

- Pain in the chest, hypochondrium (due to stagnation of blood)
- Masses in breast, masses in abdomen
- Sports injuries (impact injuries)

DOSAGE: 3–10 grams, decocted in water for an oral dose

PRECAUTIONS: Safflower should not be used by women who are pregnant, or who have heavy periods.

White Atractylodes Rhizome

ALTERNATE ENGLISH NAME: Atractylodes ovata rhizome

LATIN NAME: *Rhizoma Atractylodis macrocephalae*

PINYIN: *Bai zhu*

FLAVOR: Bitter and sweet

ESSENCE: Warm

MERIDIANS: Enters the heart, spleen, stomach, and triple warmer meridians

EFFECTS

- Strengthens the spleen and stomach, balances the abdominal organs
- Diuretic (excretes dampness, especially from lower abdominal area)
- Prevents miscarriage

INDICATIONS

- Digestive problems such as diarrhea, abdominal and epigastric distention, poor appetite
- Edema
- Restlessness, irritability
- Feeling of oppression in the chest
- Spontaneous sweating

DOSAGE: 5–10 grams, decocted in water for an oral dose; or ground into powder, or prepared in pill

White Peony Root

ALTERNATE ENGLISH NAME: None
LATIN NAME: *Radix Paeoniae alba*
PINYIN: *Bai shao yao*
FLAVOR: Bitter and sour
ESSENCE: Slightly cold
MERIDIANS: Enters the liver and spleen meridians
EFFECTS
- Nourishes the blood
- Regulates menstruation
- Nourishes the liver, balances liver function
- Reinforces yin Qi with an astringent action to stop bleeding
INDICATIONS
- Irregular menstruation, PMS, uterine bleeding, vaginal discharge
- Spontaneous sweating, night sweating
- Pain in the hypochondrium, stomach, and abdomen
- Vertigo, some types of headache
DOSAGE: 5–10 grams, 15–30 grams (large dosage), decocted in water for an oral dose

Wolfberry Fruit

ALTERNATE ENGLISH NAME: Chinese matrimony vine berry
LATIN NAME: *Fructus Lycii*
PINYIN: *Gou qi zi*
FLAVOR: Sweet
ESSENCE: Neutral

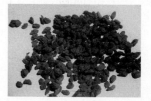

MERIDIANS: Enters the liver, kidney, and lung meridians
EFFECTS
- Strengthens the kidney, replenishes the vital essence of kidney
- Nourishes the liver
- Improves vision
- Moistens and nourishes the lung

INDICATIONS
- Deficiency in function of kidney (sometimes manifesting as weakness, particularly in the thighs and legs, sore lower back, soreness in knees)
- Blurred vision
- Dizziness
- Lung problems, particularly cough and a condition of dryness in the lung

DOSAGE: 5–10 grams, decocted in water for an oral dose

NOTES: Wolfberry fruit should not be used in cases of loose stool due to a weak spleen.

Zedoary Rhizome

ALTERNATE ENGLISH NAMES: Zedoary root
LATIN NAME: *Rhizoma Zedoariae*
PINYIN: *E zhu*
FLAVOR: Sour, sweet, slightly bitter
ESSENCE: Warm
MERIDIANS: Enters the lung, heart, and small intestine meridians
EFFECTS
- Removes heat from body
- Invigorates flow of blood
- Detoxifies
- Reduces swelling, breaks up masses

INDICATIONS
- Pain and distention in the regions of the heart and abdomen
- Stagnation of undigested food
- Menstrual difficulties, especially abnormal clotting
- Masses, tumors
- Sports injuries

DOSAGE: 5–10 grams, decocted in water for an oral dose

CONCLUSION

M ENOPAUSE is the last great energy transition or turning point of your life; it gives you an opening, a doorway to vast changes. The choices you make and the treatment you receive during this time are very important: They will determine your future.

As we've seen, the goal of TCM is to transform your whole person from the inside. Anything that enters from the outside can help a bit—making the deep and substantive changes is up to you. And, what a wonderful opportunity for transformation the energy transition of menopause offers to women. As we've discussed, the other two great opportunities are pregnancy and after childbirth. But, most Western women don't know about these special "windows for change" that can transform their health, and these special opportunities go unrecognized and unused. Taking advantage of this last great magnificent self-healing transition that is open to you takes desire, a strong belief in yourself, and patience. I believe you can do this. Just like so many of my patients, I know you have the intelligence and the sensitivity to do it. Begin to tell yourself today that you can reawaken your own healing ability and believe it. Remember that one of TCM's most important messages is "Don't wait until your house is falling down to fix it up!"

If you can take good care of yourself in every aspect of your daily life, you can make a big change, not just in the quantity, but in the fundamental quality of your Qi. Understanding the cumulative effect of all your efforts to become more healthy is one key to making this quality change. Everything is interrelated: if you focus too narrowly on just food, for instance, or just exercise, you won't unlock your full power to change.

As you progress through your menopause transition, you must be ready to deal with every aspect of your life, and make sure that every part of it contributes to your healing progress. Achieving balanced mental, emotional, and spiritual states is essential at this time, and must be nurtured through this process. Be especially mindful of this time as a gift where you can tap into that inner part of you that has always been connected to the unconditional love of the Universe.

You have now learned the importance of managing your life force or Qi. Even a small daily deposit of Qi can make your energy "checking" account grow considerably over time. Conversely, a few big energy expenditures can wipe it out. Do your best to conserve your Qi and not to waste it. When I tell my menopause patients that they are in control of their own life force, it is as if a major bell goes off in them. They suddenly comprehend that they do have this special power to transform themselves and they realize that it is they who must take responsibility for this beautiful gift. I have learned so much from the women I work with and it is my privilege to guide many of these women through what becomes one of the best times of their lives. Now I hope this ancient wisdom can help you discover your own healing power.

ACKNOWLEDGMENTS

*I*T is difficult to describe the experience of having a relationship with a master to most Western people. It's not a part of this culture. In China, having a master means a number of things, not the least of which, if you are a close enough and worthy enough student, the master will pass important knowledge obtained from his or her own masters. In some cases, this wisdom or knowledge goes back millennia. In a sense, this wisdom is inherited. It is virtually never accessible in another way or from books.

In China, there is a term for a master as well, it is *sifu*. This concept combines the idea of both master—in the sense of a great teacher, not someone who controls another—and father. In other words, the student of the *sifu*, if he or she is serious about their training, regards the *sifu* as a second father and accords him all the respect, attention, and love that a real father should receive. These are serious relationships. There is an ancient Chinese saying, "Even if you and I have only one day together as *sifu* and student, you are my father forever."

Over time, I have been privileged to work with some extraordinary masters and I would like to take this opportunity to acknowledge their phenomenal abilities and how grateful I am for their giving me secret keys to true healing. Without their assistance, I would not be able to help the people in my care in the ways that I have. I am indebted to my whole lineage for these skills and the wisdom I've been permitted to acquire.

I would like to express my appreciation to a number of people who have helped make this book a reality. I would like to thank Heather Allen for spending her time and energy working with me to shape the earlier versions of this work, which I called *Ancient Secrets: Modern Menopause*. This helped my patients gain a deeper understanding of TCM. When it became clear that menopause would be the third subject of our TCM series with HarperCollins, Pat Snyder took over the task of giving our initial materials more form and depth. We are most grateful that she pitched in so completely and helped enrich the original text further through long discussions with me, helpful additions, and insightful questions.

As always, I wish to thank my wonderful patients who have taught me so many things and helped me gain such insight into women's health problems in the west. I also want to thank my Qigong students who support my mission and work and who encourage me in this task. Thank you to Louise DiBello, Kristen Park, and others who have lent their time and talents to developing our educational materials on TCM. Thank you also to Karen Schulz for her dedication and for working so hard to ensure our graphics needs are always met. Jaime Phillips of the Eddy Foundation deserves recognition for his excellent photography; we thank the Eddy Foundation for generously underwriting the photography.

I would also like to give my deepest thanks to my writing partner, Ellen Schaplowsky. Her dedication to the mission of building bridges between the East and West and bringing the ancient wisdom of TCM to Western audiences has made this journey a lighter and happier one. It has also brought us both much joy. Without her many hours of work and determination to help me capture the appropriate words and concepts, this book would not have reached the level it has today.

To our very special editor, Ann McKay Thoroman at Harper-

Collins, we extend our sincere appreciation for her assistance and gentle guidance. To our ever-supportive and adventure-loving agent, Barbara Lowenstein of Lowenstein & Associates we again say many thanks for helping us through the intricate process of writing and publishing a book. For Ellen and for me, this would have been a difficult journey without everyone's kind encouragement and support.

TCM Personal Self-Healing Evaluation Form for Menopausal Symptoms

*H*AVE you been troubled by the following symptoms? You can use this form to track your healing progress. Make several copies so you can see how things change week to week. To start, circle the appropriate conditions. The first time you do this rate them on a scale of one to five with five being the worst. Then, check your symptoms again and rate them every week so you can chart your self-healing progress. As you begin to see your symptoms lessen in severity and duration, you will know that your body is beginning to respond to your efforts. Remember that the most important thing you can do to help yourself make a natural transition through menopause is practice the ancient Qigong movements of *Wu Ming* Meridian Therapy.

MENOPAUSAL SYMPTOMS

1. Fatigue ___	7. Chest pain ___	12. Headaches ___
2. Dizziness ___	8. Muscle tension ___	13. Stomachaches ___
3. Palpitations ___	9. Back pain ___	14. Diarrhea ___
4. Hot flashes ___	10. Loss of appetite ___	15. Constipation ___
5. Night sweats ___	11. Abdominal	16. Skin rash ___
6. Shortness of breath ___	distention ___	17. Dry mouth ___

18. Insomnia	___	22. Angry moods	___	25. Forgetfulness	___
19. Depression	___	23. Worrying	___	26. Frequent urination	___
20. Nightmares	___	24. Loss of sexual		27. Cold hands and	
21. Nervousness	___	interest	___	feet	___

	NO SYMPTOMS	MILD	MODERATE	SEVERE
Racing heart	___	___	___	___
Bone pain	___	___	___	___
Joint pain	___	___	___	___
Upset stomach	___	___	___	___
Nausea	___	___	___	___
Sweaty hands	___	___	___	___
Vomiting	___	___	___	___
Difficulty sleeping	___	___	___	___
Irritability or restlessness	___	___	___	___
Depression	___	___	___	___
Fatigue	___	___	___	___
Heartburn	___	___	___	___
Vaginal discharge	___	___	___	___
Irregular menses	___	___	___	___
Hot flashes (months)	3 mo.___	6 mo.___	12 mo.___	12 + mo.___
Average frequency	0/day___	1–3/day___	4–9/day___	10 + /day___
Night sweats	3 mo.___	1–3/day___	4–9/day___	10 + /day___
Average frequency	___	___	___	___

YOUR PHYSICAL HISTORY:

1. Heart disease: ____ heart attack ____ arrhythmias ____ angina ____ medication ____
2. Allergies: ____ food ____ other ____ fall ____ winter ____ spring ____ summer
3. High blood pressure: ____ how long ____ special diet ____ medication
4. Diabetes: ____ how long ____ special diet ____ medication
5. High cholesterol: ____ how long ____ special medication
6. Organs removed: ____ yes _____which one(s)

7. Cancer: _____ kind of cancer _____ kind of surgery _____ chemotherapy _____ radiation therapy
8. Other medical problems:
9. How many times have you been pregnant?
10. Have you ever used birth control pills? ____yes ____no. How many years? _____

YOUR MENSTRUAL HISTORY:

1. First year menstruation cycle started ____
2. Menstrual cramps: ____ none ____ before ____ during ____ after
3. Menstrual disorders: ____ early ____ late ____ irregular ____ short ____ long cycle
4. Conditions before cycle: ____ diarrhea ____ constipation ____ headaches ____ bloating
5. Vaginal discharge: ____ none ____ white ____ yellow ____ heavy
   Flow (quantity): ____ # of days ____ light ____ heavy ____ clotting ____ small ____ large
6. Color of Blood: ____ light ____ dark

YOUR MENOPAUSE HISTORY:

1. Has your menstrual cycle changed? If so, when did it begin? _____
2. What were the earliest symptomatic changes? _____
3. Are you receiving HRT or ERT therapy? _____

YOUR TCM LIFESTYLE CHECKLISTS

Check your answers and then refer back to the TCM answers in Chapter 11. Try to identify areas where your lifestyle may be compromising your health.

Eating Habits:

1. Do you eat barbecued or fried foods often? ____
2. Do you always drink ice cold drinks or ice water, particularly during your menstrual cycle? ____
3. Do you eat raw vegetables or eat at salad bars frequently? ____
4. Do you get a headache after you have a meal? ____
5. Do you experience stomach distention whenever you eat? ____
6. Do you have a stomachache after you eat, particularly after eating cold or dairy foods? ____
7. Do you always burp or pass gas after you eat? ____
8. After you eat, do you always have loose stool when you go to the bathroom? ____
9. Do you drink too much alcohol? More than two glasses a day? ____
10. Do you have food allergies? ____

Sleeping Habits:

1. Do you have difficulty going to sleep each night? ____
2. Do you wake up at the same time each night? _____ What time? ____
3. Do the same dreams recur frequently? ____
4. Do you have nightmares? ____
5. Do you experience night sweats? ____
6. Do you go to bed after midnight? ____
7. Do you eat a big meal and then go to sleep? ____
8. Do you have to take a sleeping pill or other drug to sleep soundly? ____
9. Do you get up to urinate frequently during the night? ____

Work Habits:

1. What is the average number of hours you work daily? ____ Hours worked weekly? ____
2. Do you travel a lot? ____
3. Do you work in or around high power electric areas or where there is radiation such as a microwave? _____

4. Do you work with chemicals? _____
5. Do you like your job? _____
6. Do you work under chronic stress? _____
7. Do you work straight through your day without taking a lunch break? _____
8. Do you work and eat at the same time? _____
9. Do you get along with the people you work with? _____
10. Is your work area comfortable and healthy? _____

Lifestyle:

1. Your marriage status: ____ single ____ married ____ divorced ____ widowed
2. Do you have children? _____
3. If so, do you do a lot of carpooling? _____
4. Do you do volunteer work? _____
5. Are you a member of an organization? _____More than one? _____
6. Are you always on the go? _____
7. Do you exercise? _____ Meditate _____ Yoga _____ Relaxation Exercises _____ Qigong _____Taiji _____ Other
8. Do you take time for yourself? _____

Emotions:

1. Are you depressed? _____ Do you take medication for depression? _____
2. Do you suffer from angry moods all the time? _____
3. Do you cry easily all the time? _____
4. Do you suffer from anxiety or panic attacks? _____
5. Is it hard for you to make decisions? _____
6. Do you worry all the time? _____
7. Are you under a lot of stress for continued periods of time? _____
8. Do you suffer from frequent mood swings? _____
9. Do negative events from the past continue to bother you today?_____

ABOUT THE TRADITIONAL CHINESE MEDICINE WORLD FOUNDATION

The Foundation is a nonprofit organization founded by the author Nan Lu, O.M.D., L.Ac. Its mission is to build bridges of understanding between the East and West through educational programs in Qigong, TCM, natural healing, and internal martial arts. It is dedicated to serving as the source for authentic information on TCM and Taoist Qigong.

The following programs and projects are conducted by the Foundation:

Traditional Chinese Medicine World, the Newspaper of Authentic Health and Healing

The Foundation publishes the first nationally distributed newspaper on TCM to help educate Western healthseekers about this ancient medical system and how it can enhance their well-being naturally. The newspaper reaches more than two hundred thousand readers with each issue. It is now seen in more than 75 percent of schools of acupuncture and Oriental medicine and is distributed through a private grant to more than 325 hospitals with complementary and alternative medicine centers.

The Breast Cancer Prevention Project

The Breast Cancer Prevention Project was launched in 1997. Its mission is to bring the ancient self-healing knowledge of TCM and its centuries-old experience with breast cancer and breast cancer prevention to as many women as possible. Recently, the Tamoxifen Program was added to the Breast Cancer Prevention Project. This program uses TCM principles and theories to address the root causes of the menopausal symptoms resulting from treatment with the anti-estrogenic agent tamoxifen. The Breast Cancer Prevention Project includes another HarperCollins book, *Traditional Chinese Medicine: A Woman's Guide to Healing from Breast Cancer*, a companion practice video on which Dr. Lu teaches *Wu Ming* Meridian Therapy for breast health, a series of ancient Qigong movements, an outreach program with groups like SHARE, the New York self-help organization for women with breast or ovarian cancer, and a website at www.breastcancer.com.

Women's Health Including PMS and Menopause Programs

The Foundation conducts educational programming for women's health that includes a special six-week course to help alleviate the symptoms of menopause such as hot flashes, night sweats, insomnia, irritability, and the like. TCM has been treating menopausal symptoms for thousands of years by addressing their common root causes. In fact, one famous herbal formula for hot flashes has been in use for centuries and is still used today in China. (Dr. Lu has adapted this unique classical formula for his Western menopause patients with great success. More information can be obtained by writing to the Foundation at the address at the end of this book.) Dr. Lu has extensive experience in helping Western women address their menopausal symptoms with TCM. He believes these symptoms are triggered by excess stress which, in turn, unbalances liver Qi and causes a kidney Qi deficiency.

The Dragon's Way®

The Dragon's Way is the Foundation's successful self-healing program for weight loss and stress management. It addresses the underlying factors that cause weight problems in a seven-session program. The Dragon's Way uses the best of TCM principles and theories to help individuals heal themselves and eliminate excess weight. It combines *Wu Ming* Meridian Therapy, a special eating for healing plan, and TCM herbal formulas to help participants achieve maximum benefit. To date, close to one thousand individuals have graduated from The Dragon's Way with excellent results. Participants lose, on average, twelve pounds and eight inches with The Dragon's Way. Most important are the reductions in health problems such as stress, cholesterol, high blood pressure, and the alleviation of other health issues including insomnia, food allergies, and digestive conditions, to name a few. In April 2000, HarperCollins published the second book in this TCM series with *Traditional Chinese Medicine: A Natural Guide to Weight Loss That Lasts*—Lose Twelve Pounds and Eight Inches in Six Weeks the Dragon's Way®.

The book has been so successful that it has prompted the Foundation to launch a series of one-day Dragon's Way® workshops to teach the program's *Wu Ming* Meridian Therapy Qigong movements and educate participants about the root cause of their weight problems.

ABOUT THE AMERICAN TAOIST HEALING CENTER, INC.

The American Taoist Healing Center, Inc. was founded and is under the direction of Nan Lu, O.M.D., L.Ac. The Center's mission mirrors that of the Foundation: It is dedicated to serving as the source for authentic information and training on TCM and Taoist Qigong.

PROGRAMMING

TCM Treatment

Dr. Lu maintains a practice in New York City and Bloomfield, New Jersey. He uses Taoist Qigong, acupressure, acupuncture (in New York City), moxibustion, classical Chinese herbs, and *Tunia,* or Chinese medical massage, to treat a variety of conditions. His areas of specialty include: women's health, especially breast cancer, menopause, PMS, menstrual irregularities; chronic fatigue syndrome; arthritis; hay fever; allergies; tendinitis, and sports injuries, to name a few. The focus of his practice is on preventing illness and disease, as well as helping patients heal themselves.

Wu Ming Qigong

Wu Ming Qigong is the basis of all programming at the American Taoist Healing Center and Dr. Lu's TCM practice. This unique self-healing energy system has never before been taught in the United States. It descends directly from the ancient Taoist masters Lao Tzu and Chuang Tzu. This special self-healing Qigong practice, which is easy to learn and produces results rapidly, helps students and patients connect their body, mind, spirit, and emotions for maximum healing benefit. *Wu Ming* Qigong is taught in beginner and advanced levels.

PRODUCTS

The following products have been developed by and are used by Dr. Nan Lu in his practice. They are based on classical TCM principles and theories.

- *Traditional Chinese Medicine—Ancient Wisdom for Modern Menospause—*A video session with Dr. Lu teaching eight *Wu Ming* Meridian Therapy movements. Also features a real-time practice session with Dr. Lu.
- *Traditional Chinese Medicine—A Woman's Guide to Healing from Breast Cancer—*a video with Dr. Nan Lu teaching nine *Wu*

Ming Meridian Therapy movements. Features a real-time, twenty-minute practice session with Dr. Lu.

- *Traditional Chinese Medicine—The Dragon's Way® to Weight Loss That Lasts*—A video session with Dr. Lu teaching ten *Wu Ming* Meridian Therapy movements. Also features a real-time practice session with Dr. Lu and testimonials.
- All-Natural Classical Chinese Herbal Food Supplements developed and adapted by Nan Lu, O.M.D., for a variety of health conditions, including:

    The Breast Cancer Prevention Project (BCPP) Herbal Master line of classical herbs and natural herbal teas.

    Menopause Series of Classical Chinese Herbal Food Supplements (*Green Dragon* to promote healthy liver function; *Zen Master* to help alleviate hot flashes and the discomfort of neck or lower back pain; *Imperial Qi* to strengthen kidney function; *BCPP Herbal Master IV* to boost kidney Qi; *BCPP Herbal Master I* to help strengthen digestive system function, and *CFS* to help relieve yin energy deficiency.)

- All-Natural Herbal Skin Treatment Products

    Acne Facial Masque: herbal masque helps correct underlying cause of acne;

    All Day/All Night Creme: stimulates meridians in the facial area and brings more nutrition into the face for a smoother, younger appearance;

    Silk Face Masque: a special all-natural combination of classical TCM herbs that is blended with honey; helps pull toxins from the skin and creates, smooth, fresh-looking appearance.

- Audiotapes:

    Taoist music meditations (60 minutes)

    "The Secret Behind Traditional Chinese Medicine" (60 minutes)

    "Five Element Energy Healing Meditation" (60 minutes)

ABOUT DR. NAN LU

Nan Lu, O.M.D., L.Ac., is the founder and president of the Traditional Chinese Medicine World Foundation and the American Taoist Healing Center, Inc. of New York and New Jersey. The nonprofit Foundation is the only facility of its kind dedicated to teaching *Wu Ming* Qigong in the United States. Dr. Lu is a classically trained doctor of TCM and a New York State licensed acupuncturist. His Foundation and Center are dedicated to serving as the source for authentic information on TCM and Taoist Qigong. The Foundation's mission is to build bridges of understanding between East and West in the areas of TCM, natural healing, and internal martial arts. Recently, the Foundation launched *Traditional Chinese Medicine World*, the first-ever nationally distributed newspaper dedicated to educating Western consumers and health care professionals about authentic TCM.

Dr. Lu began his training in China as a child in Taoist Qigong, TCM, and internal martial arts. Studying with several well-known, well-respected masters and doctors, he received special keys of understanding and the true essence of these ancient healing and internal martial arts. Having special knowledge passed to you is a privilege reserved for only the most advanced students. The unique healing knowledge Dr. Lu has acquired cannot be found in medical textbooks. His extensive training is the kind that ancient doctors of TCM were expected to have so that they could understand the fundamental basis of TCM—how Qi moves through the body. As a Qigong master and international martial arts champion, Dr. Lu has refined his healing practice to a very high level.

An extraordinary martial artist, Dr. Lu has won many top honors. In the fall of 1997, he competed in Argentina in the Sixth International World Cup Championship where he was named one of the top ten Taiji masters in the world. He has authored many columns for internal martial arts publications including *Pa Kua Chang* Journal, *Wushu Kung Fu,* and *Inside Kung Fu* magazines.

He is a member of the advisory group of participants for Columbia University's Center for Complementary & Alternative Medicine Research in Women's Health in a landmark study of Chinese herbs. He is also an advisory board member of the Transpersonal Psychology Association, the Hypoglycemia Support Foundation, and the USA Wushu Kungfu Federation. In New York, he works with SHARE, the self-help organization for women with breast or ovarian cancer. Through SHARE, Dr. Lu conducts a series of seminars where *Wu Ming* Qigong movements are taught to women with cancer to help them improve breast and ovarian health.

Dr. Lu holds a Doctorate in Traditional Chinese Medicine from Hubei College of Traditional Chinese Medicine, China. He has authored numerous articles on TCM and Taoist Qigong. With his "Eastern Outlook" column for *Natural Way* magazine, Dr. Lu was the first-ever columnist on TCM for a national health magazine. Dr. Lu has lectured extensively on TCM, Qigong, and self-healing in China, the United States, and England.

ABOUT ELLEN SCHAPLOWSKY

Ellen Schaplowsky has more than twenty years of experience in marketing communications work for consumer products, and in reputation management and environmental marketing. She is an executive vice president of Ruder Finn, Inc., one of the world's largest independent public relations agencies, where she founded the company's "Marketing for the Environment" Group. As part of her work in the area of environmental marketing, Ellen has served as a guest columnist for *Earth Times,* the first global newspaper on issues of the environment and sustainability that emerged from the 1992 Earth Summit in Rio de Janeiro. She is also responsible for helping create and develop America's largest litter cleanup and recycling program that annually attracts several million volunteers. For thirteen years, this program was conducted jointly by the GLAD® brand and Keep America Beautiful, Inc. It is regarded as one of the longest running partnerships in brand history.

During the early 1990s, Ellen was searching for an explanation and treatment for a complex of physical symptoms that no Western doctor seemed able to pinpoint and treat. After a number of years, she was diagnosed as having an autoimmune condition. It was at about the same time that she was introduced to the concept of Qi or "energy" and met Nan Lu, O.M.D. Ellen became Dr. Lu's patient and began a journey that would bring her deeper and deeper into TCM and its approach to self-healing and wellness. Eventually, she became a student at the American Taoist Healing Center and began practicing *Wu Ming* Qigong under the guidance of Dr. Lu.

While a patient and student, Ellen began applying her marketing communications skills to help Dr. Lu achieve his mission of serving as the authentic source for information on TCM and Taoist Qigong. At Dr. Lu's request, she became the vice president of the Center and consequently the Traditional Chinese Medicine World Foundation. In 1996, she and Dr. Lu began their writing partnership with the first-ever column on TCM for the health magazine, *Natural Way*. After more than two years of developing this column, they embarked on a more ambitious writing project, the first version of what would become *Traditional Chinese Medicine: A Woman's Guide to Healing from Breast Cancer* (Harper-Collins 1999). This collaboration marked their first book in this series of TCM works published by HarperCollins.

For more information on programs, products, and services of the Traditional Chinese Medicine World Foundation, contact:

Traditional Chinese Medicine World Foundation
396 Broadway, Suite 501
New York, New York 10013
Phone: 212. 274.1079
Fax: 212.274.9879
www.tcmworld.org
www.breastcancer.com

INDEX

Page numbers in *italics* refer to illustrations.